TRANSITIONS:
A Nurse's Education
about Life and Death

Becki Hawkins

Transitions: A Nurse's Education about Life and Death

By Becki Hawkins

Published by Lady Hawk Publishing

www.ladyhawkpublishing.com

Cover Design by Daniel Endy, Cover Photo by Hien Ngo

Layout by Launchpad Press, Cody, Wyoming

ISBN-13: 978-0-9847445-0-3

ADVANCE PRAISE FOR TRANSITIONS

"Transitions made me laugh, made me cry—happy, sad, happy, sad. Makes me wonder how I'm going to spend my time left here. After losing my husband, I like to think God took him by his hand and said, 'It's okay, come with me,' and that he went peacefully."

—Karen Hobbs

"The lessons in this book touch your heart and soul. The words reveal timeless wisdom learned from people who are getting ready to "cross over." These stories are written in such a way that you feel you are sitting right there, listening with your own ears to their voices."

—Connie Flud-Musgrave

"...Readers who have experience with Hospice, with the death of a loved one, or with their own impeding death will find many of these stories familiar and comforting. And those who have not traveled that road yet will gain insight from these stories that will be useful, sooner or later. These stories will leave you with a great appreciation for those men and women who are somehow called to nursing and ministry as their life's work."

—Steve Woodall

"This book is a collection of stories about the power of living with dying. She has a way of getting to the very heart of the last stage of life with compassion, honesty, depth, spirit, and even humor. What might seem to be a depressing subject matter is lifted up to the truth of the matter, which is that in the final goodbye, gifts abound and life is honed down to the essence of the power of love. Becki has taken that light and holds it high so we can all breathe easier, even as we contemplate that last breath."

—Robin Tilly, Martha Beck Life Coach

III

"Reading this book is a gift and a blessing. It offers a harvest of wisdom and joy, more than the average person could acquire without being in the nursing profession. "

—**Bridget Barlow,** *Currentland*

"As the baby boomers enter their twilight, Becki's wonderful book is more important than ever. Transitions allows you and your loved ones to benefit from this important information before you find yourself in a hospice situation. Through these charming stories, Becki effortlessly imparts her deep wisdom while enlightening and empowering the reader on these difficult matters."

—**Vincent Sherwood, Author of the forthcoming** *Indigo Fables*

CONTENTS

DEDICATION

This book is dedicated to my dear husband, who in the early years of my nursing career said, "You need to write about it."

Thanks, Honey!

Also, this is dedicated to all the patients and families, coworkers, supervisors: Mary Hiatt, Barbara Bilderback, and Sandee Rasnic and doctors, friends, and my own family, who helped me learn what it takes to be a nurse. My heart is full of gratitude.

And to the newspaper editor, Terry, who said, "I think we can use that in an article. Could you write one every week?" Thanks for all the encouragement over the past twenty-five years.

ACKNOWLEDGMENTS

I want to offer gratitude to the following people for their loving assistance in the creation of this book:

My God, Creator, Spirit who gave me this heart for caregiving and the desire to write.

Tom Bird for the magic he creates in his workshops, helping me to write my book in Sedona in five days! Tom, you are an old soul. Don't stop teaching us!

Thomas Hill for his excellent and compassionate editing and his patience with my concerns. And all those at Launchpad Press.

To Louis Packard for his "technical" support.

For the wise and patient webmaster, Greg, and all the others in SilverKnight.

To Daniel Endy who has helped to encourage, advise, and gently push me forward to this second edition as well as mentor me on the production of the next book.

To Hien Ngo for his gracious gift, and for allowing me to use his lovely photograph for this new cover. Butterflies always remind me of transition. We are beautiful souls here for a brief journey and then transition back Home.

For those who cheered me on from that workshop in Sedona: Dorothy, Jill, Marie, Victoria, Vinnie, Arte, Tui, RamaJon, Paul, and all the rest of you cuties!

And especially for those in my community who said, "Write it before you forget it!"

INTRODUCTION

So why write a book about all these experiences with these patients and families I've seen over the past thirty years? I think you might enjoy reading their stories. I think they matter.

I started as a nurse's aide in a nursing home, and years later became a registered nurse working in an oncology ward, and then on an outpatient oncology unit, on to hospice—home health along with hospice—and after more education became a hospice chaplain. I am now retired, so I just visit people and their families.

I've been writing a feature article titled "Beyond Statistics" for my local newspaper for years, wanting to tell others what I was experiencing with all these visits. I titled the article the way I did because I think we, in the medical profession, can often become number oriented: patient's room numbers, the number of diagnoses they have, the number of days they have been in the hospital, the number of days we think they have left to live, the number of family members in their room, etc.

What about the person in the bed: who is he or she, what is he or she feeling, what fears does he or she have, and what are the expressions on his or her face and within his or her spirit? What if we see him or her beyond all the numbers and in addition to hearing the statistics, hear them?

Some of my patients just needed their blood sugar checked and some education about diabetes, some needed chemo, and some were needing help in preparing for their soon-to-arrive passing from life.

In one article I shared the story of one patient's "near death experience." So many people came to me to thank me. Another lady came to share about her husband seeing his mother in the hospital room before he passed. She had been dead for several years. "Is that common?" she asked.

"Yes," I smiled and answered.

"Well, people need to hear about that. My husband passed in peace after he saw her. He wasn't afraid anymore," she boasted.

One particular lady saw me at a social function after that article and pulled me aside. "I want to share with you my story sometime about my 'near death experience' when I was four years old. I think others need to hear these stories. Please keep writing."

I'd helped her some with the care of her dying husband when she had first mentioned it, and I had forgotten to get back with her. So I called her a couple of days after that function and scheduled a visit.

She's just such a gracious, kind person and makes anyone and everyone feel at home and welcome in her presence. She did just that, ushering me and my husband in to see that she was in the process of packing everything up to move to a smaller home closer to family. Moving can be so emotional, especially if it is the last place you and your deceased spouse lived together. But she was remaining focused on downsizing and assessing what needed to be given away, what needed to go to family members, and what to keep for her new dwelling.

"Come sit with me at the kitchen table where there's a clear spot." She didn't hesitate to start sharing. My dear husband loves her like I do and didn't move a muscle while she talked.

"I was four years old. I had polio and was very ill. I was in the hospital in a long ward with other children who also had polio. I had a high fever and I was in terrible pain. My father was with me, trying to comfort me. All of a sudden I was out of my body floating up. I could see the nuns walking up and down that corridor and then I was surrounded in the most wonderful warmth and light, filled with peace, pain gone, and so much love surging throughout my little body. I saw my father and his concern and the nurses running toward my body on that bed. Then I was back on that bed and the horrible pain returned. When I tried to tell my father about what had happened, he told me not to tell anyone because it was just a dream. Years later when the near death experience books started appearing in bookstores and in the news, I thought, 'That's what happened to me. I knew it wasn't a dream!'

"I know it didn't last long, but it was long enough. I am not afraid to die because of that. You can't find the words to describe that peace and love you feel. But I hope that sharing my story might help someone else. And it's validating to be heard."

As one lovely soul once shared with me, no matter who we are, where we live, or where we go to church (or not), we are one human family. We are spiritual beings having these human experiences for a very short time so that we can learn to love.

They remind me that it's all so brief, so fragile, and so very precious, that we are all in transition. We cannot judge where others are in their journey, but we can peek at our own.

So, as you read these stories, let them bless you in any way they are speaking to your heart.

Peace,

Becki

Author's Note: Many of the people in these stories are still living in my hometown. So, I changed the names, and sometimes the directions to their homes, and if I said they had a cat, it may have been a dog. Privacy is premium in a small town.

PART ONE
THE EARLY YEARS

CHAPTER 1

MY INTRODUCTION TO CAREGIVING

Annie was only about four feet tall and had a husband about 4'2", and they had moved into the nursing home due to their forgetfulness and lack of family to help them. I thought they were the cutest little people on the face of the Earth. One day I caught Annie in the bathroom with a flyswatter stirring the water in the toilet bowl. "Annie, what on earth are you doing?" I asked. Well, I'm stirring up these brown beans before they burn." The tone in her voice gave me the sense that she also wanted to say, "What else would you think I'm doing?"

Her sweet hubby, John, just stood and stared at her like he hoped there would be cornbread to go with the beans.

Then there was Bertie who would whistle up and down the corridor while scooting along in her wheelchair. She loved bananas and would stop every so often and ask another client, "Hey, Buddy, got a banana on ya?" When Santa showed up at Christmas it was a banana he pulled out of his toy bag for Bertie. She was the happiest client in the room.

One other lady was always singing and making up the songs as she rolled along in her wheelchair pushing anyone who got in her way. "Dear Lord, please say to me that you are coming soon. And don't pay attention to me singing out of tune." She would tell the little guy in front of her, "Move on, brother. Move on. Time's not standing still for anyone. And I need to get to the dinner room before I die. I'd like to go with a full stomach." And then she would laugh until her dentures nearly fell into her lap.

Then there was the little blind gentleman who would take all his clothes off and wander into the hallway and sometimes into the room down the hall. Screaming started coming from the lady who thought he was trying to get in bed with her. Her alarming sounds would fill the east wing, "Help, there's a naked man in my room! HELPPPP!!!" And she would start poking him with her umbrella and then he would start screaming. Then the other women in that wing would come out and holler, "Where's a naked man?"

One evening I was staying a little later than my assigned shift time to visit with Mrs. Smith as long as possible. The nurse in charge told me she was not doing too well and they didn't expect her to make it through the night. When I got back to work the next morning I hurried to her room. The door was closed. I opened it with caution to see that all Mrs. Smith's belongings were gone. I closed the door and headed down the hall. Jane saw me and rolled out to greet me. "Becki, you mustn't cry about Mrs. Smith. She's not having to worry about whether or not someone's going to keep force-feeding her. She does not have to worry about getting that cold or hot shower twice a week by someone's who in a hurry."

I looked at her and said, "But she's gone. And what if she was alone when she died?"

"Yes, she's gone. And it doesn't matter anymore if she was alone or not. She's not alone anymore. And you mustn't be sad for her. She's just gone from her body. Her spirit is safe."

I turned the corner and sat down in the mop closet. I pulled my knees up close to my chest and cried like a baby for five minutes. I thought, "I don't think I'm as sad for Mrs. Smith as I am for me."

4

CHAPTER 2

A SURPRISE LESSON IN NURSING SCHOOL

When I was in nursing school I was visiting a patient in the psych ward in the veterans' hospital. He was due to have surgery the next day for lung cancer. They were going to remove as much of the tumor as they could. His other diagnosis was a manic-depressive disorder. Today we call it bipolar disorder. He had long reddish hair that was braided and hanging down his back with the curlier gray hairs along the side of his temples poking out. They dared to look like they couldn't be tamed into that braid, almost a Willie Nelson look-alike. He was in his manic phase then, and I first met him racing up and down the hallway stating as loud as he could, "Give the Lord all your money. Give the Lord all your praise. Bless his Name. Give Oral Roberts some too. I'm going to Heaven tomorrow. Saints protect us. Bless the Lord, oh my soul."

There were nine beds lined up in his ward where he slept. My job was to trim his toenails before his surgery the next morning. I couldn't believe it. I was scheduled to graduate in the upcoming semester and I had to trim a guy's toenails!! "What a waste of time," I thought. What would I learn from that?!

5

I had him sit down in a high-backed chair—a feat in itself—and got his warm, sudsy water all fixed up for him and the nail trimmers retrieved from the nurse in charge (no one was allowed to have them in their bedside table drawer). Then he started singing and shouting all over again: "Going to Heaven in the morning to see my Jesus. Yes, I am. Lord, bless the little nurse cleaning my feet for my Heaven arrival."

One of the other nine roommates entered the room. He was schizophrenic (I found out later) and peered around and looked at both of us. My patient spoke up, "Hey, buddy, where you been? What you been doing? I'm getting my feet and toenails all cleaned up by this little nurse lady." Then out of the blue the guy walks over to my patient and hits him right in the middle of his forehead with his fist!

I scrambled under the first available hospital bed. I started screaming and shouting myself this time. "Help! Help! Somebody help me in this room!"

Two orderlies come running in. They took a look at my patient and the other fellow with his fists still all tight and they hauled him away.

My supervisor/instructor came into the room and looked under the bed where I was hiding. "Becki, you can come out now."

My patient starting shouting and testifying, "God saved me. God sent this little nurse lady in here to clean my toenails and she ended up saving my life by screaming for help! God bless America. Give all your money to Oral Roberts. Give God all the glory. I'm going to Heaven in the morning."

Back at the classroom in school, my teacher asked me, "Becki, did you learn anything today?"

"Yes, ma'am," I nodded with embarrassment. Then when I got the courage I asked her if I could go see my little fellow before his surgery in the morning. She agreed if I got permission from the nurse in charge of his unit.

So, with approval I got up extra early and went in to see him

6

before his scheduled surgery. He smiled at me and said, "Thank you for being there for me, missy." He was drugged with a little pre-med for surgery and was so much calmer.

"Would you like for me to pray with you before I go?" I humbly asked.

"Yes, little lady, I would," he replied.

When I came back after my classes that afternoon to check on him I couldn't find what room he was in. I went to his unit and asked his nurse in charge. She simply looked at me and shook her head and then took me aside. "I'm sorry to tell you but he died in surgery."

Driving home that evening I couldn't help but think, "He wasn't that delusional after all."

CHAPTER 3

NEW NURSE

Seven years later I was able to go to nursing school, and the first job I had was on the oncology floor at a large hospital. I had the same feeling that came over me when I first went to work at the nursing home. I was so glad to be there every day, and I was always so very tired when I went home. The education for me was all that filled the hours in between! At first I couldn't believe they were paying me! That wore off.

Mr. Smith was in a room in the pod of five rooms where I was working that night. And there were five really sick patients to be seen. Someone needed packed red blood cells, another patient needed chemotherapy after we had provided instructions to him about the drugs and their side effects, and yet another patient needed IV antibiotic for an infection due to the low white blood cell counts from the chemo he had received a week or so before.

And then there was this fellow in Room 9705. He was hunkered down deep into his blankets and chilling and shaking like his bed had grown legs and was leaving and taking him with it. I peeked just under the covers and whispered his name, "Mr. Smith? Are you doing okay under all these blankets? I need to check your temperature and see if you are ready for some more Tylenol."

He peeked out and said, "Nurse Lady, would you please bring me another blanket with that fever medicine? Don't matter if my fever is up or down at this moment. What I need is relief. I feel likes my skin is going to crawl off me."

I got his meds, headed back to his room, and saw him out of the bed, now on his knees praying like there was no tomorrow. "My Lord Jesus, my Sweet Savior, hear me now, I pray. I know you know me by name. I know you know my situation down here, and I'm asking, dear Lord, for you to please help these doctors and nurses know how best to help me. I ask, Lord, too, please help these poor folk who are in this hospital to have what they needs, too, as I can hear them troubled families crying on their way to the elevator, and I can feel in my soul the anxious hearts that are trying to help their loved ones in these here beds. Sweet, sweet Lord, we trust you with all this here suffering as we don't know how else to handle it. You be knowing best for us and the timing. Just give us the strength to hang on as long as we're suppose to and help us not to be afraid of the time when we needs to lay down our worn out bodies and come on home to you."

Then I helped him crawl back up into his bed, covered him, raised the head of his bed, gave him the meds he needed, and leaned in close. I kissed his feverish brow and said, "Mr. Smith, I'm sure the Lord heard your earnest prayer. I know you know him on a first-name basis. We will do all we can here to make you comfortable, and we too will pray for God to do the rest. You rest and sleep and keep on trusting." I can still see that sweet gentle man praying for others.

Within the hour he started having seizures that seemed to go on forever. His doctor stood on one side of the bed and I was on the other side, with the aide beside me touching me on the arm to comfort me as the tears ran down my face. We had given him the anti-seizure meds in his IV and waited. He stopped having the awful seizures. He smiled and then he stopped breathing. Honoring his request not to bring him back to life, we just stayed with him and I patted him like he might still be aware. "Go in peace, Brother Smith."

The supervisor, knowing I was still learning, helped me with the rest of the patients that evening. Then she took me aside to ask me if I was okay. I told her yes, but that I was sad.

"Sad? For him?" she questioned.

"Yes, well, and sad for me," was all I could get out.

She nodded.

I went home one evening after an especially long shift and was about to tell my dear husband about how I had been challenged one way and another, learning how to balance out all this suffering I saw with the occasional good news that someone got to go home not needing any more chemo. He stopped me, "Please don't tell me any more stories. Could you just write them down? Maybe that would help you." Bless him.

I crawled into the shower and let the warm water hit me in the face and then sat on the shower floor. I cried and cried and asked God to please give me strength to be able to help those patients and their families and not make my family crazy in the process. Then I dried off and got out the ink pen and paper.

That's how my career in writing began.

CHAPTER 4

TELL ME EVERYTHING

L isa wasn't much older than me when she was diagnosed with cancer just days before her admission to our unit. Her doctor asked me to bring in the info sheets for her chemo that we would begin that evening. I went to the med room to gather my supplies: chemo gown, chemo gloves, and the syringes with the meds to help limit the nausea and to help keep her calm. Plus, there was the chemotherapy itself.

I went in to check on her and found her eight-year-old son piled up in bed with her. She held him tightly. Her parents were on the visiting couch with them watching and holding one another. They were too frightened to speak and also very respectful of the way she would talk frankly to her son. They were not trying to tell her how to do any of it. They just were trying to be there for her.

"It's okay, baby," she told him as she stroked his shiny brown hair. "I feel better since I cried. And we're going to fight this and be strong while we are fighting! Right?!"

"Yes, Mama. We will be strong for you."

Then he went back to his grandparents and asked them if they would take him to get a Dr. Pepper. The three of them left as I began putting the IV supplies on the bedside table.

She didn't waste time pulling herself up in bed, announcing, "Becki, I want you to tell me everything about these drugs—all the good they are going to do and all the side effects I can expect. I always want the truth from you. Do you understand me?" she said with a smile.

"Yes. And I agree to do that," I replied. I loved being the nurse. I hated the chemo. My wise supervisor told me later when I told her about my feelings that it wasn't abnormal to feel that way. I was glad to hear it. The only other opening for a job was in obstetrics and I never did too well with those dear women and all that screaming.

And so we began.

I drove home that evening thinking, "Is there an okay age to have to go through this?" No. I don't care if the patients are sixteen or 106. If they get the news that they need chemo and radiation, it's still hard news to take at first. I think it was that she was close to my age that got me.

She never did say she was quitting or giving up the fight when the doctors told her the chemo wasn't working. She went on to another state for a bone marrow transplant and did fair for a while. Again her son and her parents totally supported her. But the bone marrow transplant failed. She decided to come home to be near family and friends during her last days. She died with grace and dignity and gratitude after all she had been through. I wasn't doing too well with the news.

One of the more experienced nurses sat down with me in the nurses' lounge and said quietly, "You need to understand something. We save some and we lose some, and we do the best we can following the doctors' orders and the patients' wishes. Just because they die sometimes doesn't mean it was anything you or I did wrong. The cancer killed them. I know you're young, and that may be hard to hear at your age. But, Sugar, we don't live forever, and no one ever got a written note from God that everyone's suppose to live to be eighty

12

years or more. That's what is so hard for many people, when they think that they're being cheated out of their right to more days and years and anniversaries and birthdays and graduations. It just isn't so, my dear. Our most important day is today, this day. We have to live and enjoy where we are, knowing that it's all very precious and very fragile, and there's no guarantee that there's tomorrow. So you need to go home tonight and kiss your family before you go to bed and bless the good Lord when your feet hit the floor in the morning when you get up. If you wake to a new day, then don't waste it. You need to honor the footprints you are making while you are here."

I heard her and did understand, somewhat, what she was trying to tell me, but it took many more years and many more patients before I fully came to grips with anyone's death.

CHAPTER 5

GOD'S SHOULDERS

I was working on an oncology floor in the mid '80s, and I had a patient who was not doing well. There were benches in the pod that lined the walls, placed for family members to come out and sometimes rest or just regroup. One of the patient's wives was sitting there listening one day to the noise coming from one of the rooms, the room where one patient of mine was taking a turn for the worse. His brother was ranting and raving with all his angst and his frustration. "Why aren't they doing something else?" Why isn't this medication working? Why is God letting him die?" The young man's mother spoke, "Son, don't question God. We aren't supposed to do that."

The lady on the bench saw me come out of the room with my own angst. She motioned for me to come to the visitors' lounge. She carried such a peace with her wherever she was. It wasn't a chore to follow her. She said, "Sit down with me a minute. I want to tell you something. I heard that young man's questioning God about his brother and his mother telling him not to do that. We all need to know that God doesn't care if we question Him. God knows our hearts are full of questions and pain and fear. God's shoulders are big enough to take all we direct His way. Now, rest assured, I'm not going to go in there and try to line that dear family out, but I will pray for their peace to come in the midst of their painful time."

"But what about me? Should I stay silent, too? I feel so sorry for them, and I can't do any more than I'm doing. The cancer isn't responding to the chemo," I said, wringing my hands and running them through my hair.

"Becki, darlin', I see your pain and concern as you go in and out of these doors. You must stop trying to be God, sweetheart. God knows His business. Your job is to do exactly what you are doing. You are here to give the medications the physician orders, educate about the chemo and radiation and their side effects, give pain medicine as the doctor dictates, help with the nutritional needs, let the respiratory therapy folk know when they are to get up here, call the chaplain if needed. But then you walk away and lay it down and go home to your family and your time.

"If you go on trying to carry all this in your heart, you're going to lose your love of nursing and helping. You do what you can, and then you trust God with the rest.

"Look out that window there. We are twelve stories up. See all those people driving down that busy street? Each one of them are having troubles all their own, whether their husband done up and left them, or the bank is calling about a late payment on their house, or their job is looking like it might end pretty soon. All of us, child, are learning our lessons. This is Earth School. We are here to learn and to love. The sooner you know this without a doubt and put it to practice, the sooner you going to breathe easier every day you step off that elevator to clock in to go back to work here.

"Now, go on back out there. I've done gone to preachin'. I pray for you every day, and I won't stop."

I wasn't old enough or smart enough to really hear what she said then. But I hear her now, and I'm listening better.

15

CHAPTER 6

I SEE YOU

I went to see a movie with my family a couple of years ago. It was *Avatar*, and these people in the movie were able to look at each other and see each other emotionally as well as physically. So when one would look at another they might say, "I see you." And they would REALLY mean it.

I was working the late shift—evening shift, that is—at the time, and I was giving IV pain medication to one of my patients, Mr. Jones. He was a nice minister with a nasty cancer. Most of the time he was quiet and didn't say much. I sat down on the foot stool next to his bed to slowly push the medication into his tubing so as not to cause any unwanted side effects if it went into his vein too fast. I had turned my head downward to peek at the urine output in his catheter bag and sighed without realizing it.

"I see you, and I hear you," he whispered.

I jumped and was startled. "Oh, I'm sorry. I didn't mean to disturb you, Mr. Jones."

I was horrified that I must have sounded so unprofessional.

"You are human. You are tired, and I sense an even deeper level

16

to that sigh. You are dealing with something that is in your heart and not just in your fatigue."

"Mmm, you are right." I hesitated.

"Me, too," he continued.

"Really?"

"I thought I had enough faith to whip this cancer. I thought that if I just believed in the power of Jesus' healing touch that I'd be home now celebrating. I've been rethinking this. Don't misunderstand me. I believe Jesus can heal anyone, anywhere, anytime. But I'm also just beginning to know that my God loves me just the same if he cures me or if he doesn't cure me. I may live until I'm 110, but if I die soon, either way, I'm heading to my eternal home.

"I've been clinging to this belief system of having it just one way in my head. If you believe enough, if your faith is big enough, you can know a total healing. But in my mind, my faith couldn't be any stronger. And to think that for years I've thought that those who died preaching about their faith in being healed just didn't have the right faith or enough faith. Well, it makes me so sad. I don't know what you are dealing with tonight. I do want you to know God loves you. And he cares about what's in your heart. I want to encourage you to trust that no matter what happens. And I want you to pray for me as you walk these halls, as well as for all of us, that we too can trust our God and His will with our lives.

"If I go home, I plan to write a brand new sermon. I think I'll title it 'Rest Assured.'"

I didn't worry about my unprofessional sighing that evening anymore. That dear man, who had so much going on in his head and his body and his heart, heard me and blessed me with his wise words. I'm still working on that sermon in my own head.

It reminded me that I can never judge another's faith or lack of faith. There's healing beyond what we can see with our human eyes.

CHAPTER 7

IT'S NOT YOUR FAULT

In the very early part of my oncology nursing days, I was caring for Eli, a young man in his twenties. He had a rare blood disease that his oncologist was trying to eliminate with aggressive chemo. He was movie star beautiful for now, thick black shiny hair, and a movie star beautiful wife who loved him beyond measure. Often I had to coax her out of his bed to do a dressing change to a deep wound near his spine. We had to pack it with sterile iodine-soaked ribbons of gauze and cover it with sterile pads and then tape it.

They went to a church that taught about believing enough to claim healing and not letting anyone say a negative word that might mess up the claim. Two men from their church "stood guard" outside his room. My patient said they were there to help keep negative people or thoughts away from him so he could build up his faith. One of the seasoned nurses wanted to drag them out to the elevator and pitch them in it or worse. The supervisor told her to ignore them. Boy, were they lucky!

One evening I found him in his bathroom on the cold floor praying his heart out, pleading with God "for the faith required." I gently tapped his shoulder and said, "Eli, you need to get back in bed. I promise you, God hears you just as good in your bed. Your blood counts are so low and we need to protect you from any infection. I don't know if this floor is sterile."

I got him back in bed, and he took my hand. "Please pray for me to get well. My wife and I want me to go home and we want to do God's work and we want to have enough faith in that."

All I could eek out was, "Please, God, be with Eli and Mary." My pager went off and I nearly ran out of that room knocking one of the soldier boys off his post.

I was thinking about them a couple of evenings later as I was driving to work. The notion of "having enough faith" was a big topic. When I arrived one of the nurses told me that Eli had left the hospital "AMA," against medical advice, the day before. He said they were going to Florida. He said it was showing he had the faith required by leaving the hospital and declaring this healing was taking place. I sat dumbfounded for a few minutes trying to take it all in and grasp the enormity of what had just taken place. The seasoned nurse left the room cursing a blue streak.

One evening, about a month later, I was writing in a patient's chart and Mary showed up. She was alone. Eli had died within two weeks of arriving in Florida. She felt like it was her fault because her faith wasn't strong enough. Down the hall the seasoned nurse stomped away from us. One of the other nurses grabbed Mary and pulled her into the nurse's report room and said, "Listen, sweetie, you didn't kill your husband. The cancer killed him. And whether you stayed or you left probably in this case didn't make a whole lot of difference. He wanted to go. You wanted to be with him. You did not cause his death."

Mary looked unimpressed, like she had heard those words before but couldn't absorb them. We loved on her, encouraged counseling, and waved her good-byes as she walked away.

I hope she was able to find new faith.

CHAPTER 8

ONE BRAVE SOLDIER

Mr. Brown didn't really fit on his bed even though we had gotten the extra long one up there before he was admitted. My supervisor warned me to not take anything that he said too personally. She said he was an old veteran who cursed and swore and liked young nurses.

His doctor allowed him to smoke a cigar with supervision for about five minutes every day. He was dying. And, besides, he tended to chew on his cigars more than he actually smoked them.

When I went to make my introduction and do my assessment of him he whistled and roared in his gruff, gravel, big ole' voice, "Well, hello, Sunshine! Where have you been all my life?"

I would normally have been entertained but couldn't help but notice the blood on his sheet. He was oozing blood slowly from all over his body. You never forget that smell.

I excused myself and went back to get the dressing cart and returned to redress all these bleeding sites. His skin was thin and black and blue and red and purple with the appearance of his insides trying to escape through his skin. I had never seen anything of the sort before—and haven't since.

"Just wrap me up some more, Cupcake. It'll be fine. And, when you get through seeing your other patients come back in here, we'll share that stogie in my bedside table drawer. Doctor gave me permission, so don't get all holy and tell me I can't have it. Besides, I want to look at you some more and tell you war stories." And then he roared a laugh and smiled from ear to ear, hollering as I exited the room, "What do you have to say about that?

"I even bet we could get a snort of whiskey—or how about Scotch? Yeah, that's what we need. Call up that nutrition lady who always wants me to be drinking more fluids and tell her I want some smoky Scotch! Oh, that'll get her goat!!"

I lost it. I couldn't help but smile as I was pointing my finger at him.

"No Scotch tonight. We'll fix you up with a chew on your cigar just because your doctor said so, but he didn't say a thing about Scotch!" I tried to say with a controlled voice as I backed out the door.

"Leave that door open a crack. I'm not wanting to be by myself in here without being able to see an escape in case I need one," he firmly stated.

I wasn't able to leave him alone too much that evening with all his bleeding. I needed to reapply the dressings frequently and give him another two units of packed red blood cells.

His doctor decided that the blood transfusions weren't really helping him all that much, so he talked to him. "Sure, Doc. You know your stuff. We know how it is. You've done all you can. You're a good soldier, Doc. I'm ready to meet this enemy head-on."

Some of the employees thought the doctor was out of line by giving that patient a chew on his cigar. I even heard that someone snuck him in some Scotch one evening. These days it would never happen—okay, well, maybe. But, at that time, for that patient, I was tickled that he got his wishes.

21

CHAPTER 9

THE POWER OF TOUCH

I was working in a smaller big city hospital in the outpatient oncology department. We had been giving Jim chemo for a big cancer in his brain. He made me smile every time he got off that elevator with his wife. He was over six feet tall and weighed over 250 pounds (in the beginning), and his face was a rosy color with a huge smile. He always wore bib overalls, a plaid short-sleeved cotton shirt, and big lace-up boots. Jim's wife, Betty, followed him with pride and said less than he did.

"Good morning, girls! Who wants to draw my blood today?" he beamed like it was an honor.

"I will! It's my turn. Come over here and sit in this recliner and we'll get started," I said eagerly.

The great thing was how large and giving his veins were. The scary thing was that after I got the blood in the tube, white matter rose to the top of the blood. I had never seen that before meeting him. The other nurse working there, who had been my mentor when I first starting my career, told me that it was fat in his blood. She said, "Becki, we aren't worrying about that at this point. We're just trying to slow down his tumor's growth. He knows, but he still stays positive and cheerful."

So, every week he came for his lab work and his chemotherapy for four weeks and then he would have a week off. Never once did I not see him smile getting off that elevator. But, as time passed, he quit wearing his lace-up boots and instead wore his house shoes. His overalls were hanging on him. Nonetheless, he kept showing up though with his positive attitude.

He was admitted to the hospital for a blood transfusion and IV antibiotics for an infection he couldn't get rid of with oral antibiotics. I headed up the back stairs to go check on him one afternoon after we had finished seeing patients. I peeked into his room to see if he was sleeping. He turned and smiled. "Come on in here. How is everyone downstairs? Look at this mess I'm into up here. They are giving me blood and medicine in this arm and now they're wantin' to give me some drink to help me gain some strength and weight back. That stuff tastes really bad! I don't think too many folk that need it are going to like it. They better come up with something a mite different." His wife grinned and shook her head.

"So, how are you feeling?" I asked as I sat on the edge of his bed and took his hand. His wife got up and excused herself to go down to the cafeteria.

"Well, to tell the truth, I'm a little concerned, but my faith is strong, and I know my Lord will see me through this, one way or the other. You can't throw your faith out the window if everything isn't going exactly like you want it to. God has never turned his back on me and I'm not turning my back on him. And, truly, I think these doctors have given me and the wife some more time. But, before I forget it, I want to tell you what a joy it has been for me to come see you girls all this time, even though it was for treating my cancer. I looked forward to every visit and getting to talk to those other patients and their families.

"The thing I want to say is this. Thank you for treating me like I was the most important patient you had every visit. Now I know, I know you girls treat everyone of us like that. But no one but my wife has ever touched my hand with as much compassion as you girls do. Some of the kinfolk have acted like I have a contagious disease, and act like they might catch my cancer from me, if they hugged me or shook my hand. Isn't that the strangest thing? Bless their hearts. They don't know no better. Somebody ought to write a book for the public to have a better idea of how to treat their friends or neighbors or family who has cancer."

I leaned over and with as much gentleness as possible, hugged him, and kissed his flushed cheeks. He smiled from ear to ear. "Aw, Becki, thanks. Thanks for everything." I nodded and said, "No, thank you. You have been such a gift to us downstairs. You bring such positive energy everywhere you show up! You have blessed us and the other patients. God's love is beaming out of your whole body."

"Aw, Becki, shucks. Don't go on like that. It's embarrassing." He grinned from ear to ear with a brighter red face now.

We prayed together and I slowly made my way back down the stairs. "Thank you, God, for Mr. Smith. Help us remember to show your love like he does. Help us remember to not be afraid to pat a hand, touch a shoulder, give a Holy Hug when appropriate. Amen."

CHAPTER 10

THE LANDSCAPE

I rolled up on my stool next to Fred to start eyeballing his arms for a suitable vein to give him his chemo. He had been coming in for monthly treatments for several months now. His color this visit was between yellow and an orange-brown. He was tall and thin, but stronger than when we first met.

Today, he brought us fresh tomatoes and cucumbers. He chatted with me as I gathered supplies and then wasted no time in saying what he wanted to say: "The landscape is different now."

"What landscape?" I questioned and then focused on taping the IV line down while trying to avoid too much hair on his arm.

"At home. Before I started all this radiation and chemo and lab work and scans and bone marrow tests, I went for walks along the shoreline of the lake where we live. I was thinking about the stock market, international trade, politics, commodities, annuities, how many miles I could walk before heading to the office, controlling my son's future from our home to his dorm room..."

"Oh," I glanced up again, "tell me how it's different."

"The sunlight glistens on the water's waves like crystal beads.

The Canadian geese seem to be thinking over staying here instead of flying south. My sense of smell is picking up the mixture of decaying leaves, last night's rain, and years of pine needles and wildflowers. I hear my feet crunching leaves and rotting wood pieces from fallen old oaks recycling themselves back into the earth. I sat on a log yesterday and watched worms, rollie-pollies, and ants, and could hear bees and flies, and caught the sunlight through the trees throwing a dragonfly's iridescent color scheme my way."

"Cool!" I smiled and then patted his arm.

"I'm trying not to beat myself up too much about thinking I was really in control of everything in my life. What a joke. I would have never in a million years chose cancer. But, it's a threshold that's given me a fuller relationship with my son and wife that perhaps I'd never gained otherwise...done already? See you next month."

I drove the hour-long commute home that evening reflecting on what he had said to me. I went out and sat in the middle of my flower bed and watched some ducks land on my grandpa's pond. But within five minutes, I was thinking about laundry that needed to be done, weeding the flowerbeds before mulching them, and what to fix for supper.

I smiled as I got up and thought out loud, "Oh well, maybe you'll get better at 'landscaping' with time."

CHAPTER 11

RESPECTED BOUNDARY LINES

A s the years rolled on I discovered that I could never guess what would be coming my way each day.

The previous shift's nurse knew I was still learning and didn't want to frighten me.

"Okay, kiddo, listen up and put your brave face on," she said.

"This lady in Room 10, Mary, has really had a rough morning. Her lungs started filling up fast, but we've got her fairly stable for a while. You have to keep a close eye on her, okay? She knows she's dying. Her sister, Bea, knows she's dying. But they're sort of taking care of one another and dancing all around it. You pay attention to them, and you'll learn a thing or two."

I decided to check on her first. "Good afternoon, I've heard you had a busy morning but that you're breathing easier now. What do you think?" I asked while looking for signs of distress or discomfort.

"Better," was all she managed with a weak smile. She reached for my hand, trying to display her courage.

Bea motioned for me to step outside the room with her. "My sister's been uncomfortable all day, and she's not the type to wake

27

up complaining unless she is in horrific pain. We both know she doesn't have long, and I want her to be comfortable. After that bad spell this morning, she told me she knew the end was near."

Tears were making their way down her face.

"We are sisters, you know, and I am the oldest. I won't leave her tonight. Her husband is exhausted and home with their toddlers. We live close to each other, and I've been with her through all of this."

She ended the discussion by reaching for my hand. Must be a family trait. Nevertheless, her unspoken statement was clear. She was in charge and her invisible boundary lines were drawn and respected.

As the evening progressed, I watched her monitor all activities in the room. Only with her sister's approval were visitors allowed, and only five minutes at a time. If privacy became an issue, everyone was ushered out. When the patient asked for some face cream, Bea made the call to another family member. Oil of Olay was delivered and was gently applied to her flushed cheeks. Mary requested Coke for dinner and that was all. That too was respected by all the nurses and visitors.

Mary gave Bea permission to be sad; Bea gave Mary permission to go.

After administering some IV pain medication, Bea spoke quietly, "Our parting is only temporary. We get that. We are sisters forever and beyond this disease, this hospital, this earth. We are doing our best to be brave, but it's hard. Will you please pray for us as you continue your rounds this evening?"

"Yes," I nodded.

I did. And I called both of my sisters the next day.

CHAPTER 12

THE SEVENTY-FIFTH WEDDING ANNIVERSARY

I had the honor of officiating in a wedding one summer. The darling couple, looking like Brad Pitt and Angolina Jolie, is still in that star-struck stage when they look at each other.

At the time my husband and I were celebrating forty years of marriage, and he said he didn't remember that star-struck stage.

I helped care for Annie and Bill in 1971. They had outlived all four of their children. They were frail but mentally strong, and tolerated my questions. They were celebrating their seventy-fifth wedding anniversary. I had never met anyone who had attained such a status.

They sat in side-by-side, handmade, oak rockers. She was a stout woman with her hair combed back tightly into a low-sitting bun roll that was a silver, grayish color. Her dress looked right out of the '40s, and so did her black lace-up shoes. Her stockings were rolled up above her knees and tied with a piece of fabric. I'd seen that before on my grandmother, so that didn't shock me.

He was very thin with wire-rimmed glasses hanging off the end of his long, pointed nose, was nearly totally deaf, and had thinning white hair cut really short above the ears and way up the nape of his neck. He had on bib overalls and a short-sleeved cotton plaid shirt with a hankie stuffed in the front bib pocket. Both of them were just too cute for words, looking like a Norman Rockwell calendar picture.

"So, which one of you deserves the biggest crown in this marriage?" I asked them.

They looked at each other and grinned, then pointed at each other with "He does!" and "She does!"

"Mother, you talk to her. My teeth are loose, and I'm clacking too much," he said.

"All right, come sit here close to me on this little foot stool and let me tell you what everybody always asks us: 'How'd they stay married that long?'

"You have to understand that when me and Father got married there wasn't any question of not staying married. His dad gave us a section of land to get us started with, a little ole' four-room house, an outhouse, a sagging faded barn, a milk cow, a mule, and a sway-backed horse, a sow, and a few chickens. There was work to do to survive. We were a team. It was hard times, and there wasn't much time for fussing 'cause we were so gol-dern tired at the end of the day. I think we were just glad we'd made it another day.

"We were blessed, both of us, with parents who were godly and gave us good examples about how to raise a family. We weren't so serious every minute, though. We did raise four kids. You know, life's uncertain, and I think we are both trying to figure out why we're still here and our kids are all gone now. We leave it with God. We think we must still be here for a reason. Maybe it's to tell you young folk our story, who knows?

"Father, what do you want to tell her?" she hollered over in his good ear.

"Don't go to bed mad, don't spend money you don't have, find something to laugh at every now and then, go to a barn dance and dance with your wife like she's the best looking woman there. Remember, if one of ya needs to be in the barn tinkering with something longer than usual, or if the other one of ya needs to be fussing alone in the kitchen way after supper dishes are done, let 'em alone," he hollered back, and then slumped back into his padded rocker, eyes closed. That wore him out!

"Oh, yes, it does a couple good if you pray for each other. We still do that," she added. "And remember, a vow is a vow."

That was it.

They both fell asleep, exhausted from our chat.

Lucky me.

I've never met anyone since who has been married that long. My husband says God has a sense of humor and He's keeping us married no matter what.

CHAPTER 13

PROMISE ME

I was in my teens when my sister and I began babysitting for Laura's two very young daughters, Linda and Lacey. The youngest little cutie had curls and was still very attached to her pacifier.

My sister turned out to be the best sitter, since I was more interested in driving fast and chasing boys back then and moved up to a more lucrative job, working at the Dairy Queen.

But we were always in touch with Laura through the years. In a small town you grow up with the town. She was maybe five feet tall, tiny features, beautiful curly blondish locks, big expressive brown eyes, and impeccable taste in her clothes, shoes, and bags. And her personality matched all that.

Years passed and the girls were grown and on their own. I was seeing hospice patients at the time she called.

Her dear husband was dying and he had decided he wanted his hospital bed in the living room, at an angle facing the television, which he wanted on day and night, and he wanted the pets to be able to get up on the bed and for their granddaughter to be able to crawl up there as well.

If anyone turned off the TV, he would wake up with, "Hey, who did that? Can't you see that I'm watching that show!?"

His lovely wife, Laura, was cleaning and cooking, nursing and entertaining. He just didn't have much time left with such an aggressive cancer.

"Promise me," he pleaded with her, "you'll keep me comfortable."

"Of course, you know I will," she replied.

And that was our goal in keeping him home with his doctor's help. No one could have been a better nurse than she was. With energy only someone with immeasurable love can have, she tirelessly gave her all in keeping her promise.

I kept in touch with her over the next few years and one day received another call from her. "I have a rare cancer, but I'm fighting it. They told me I'm terminal, but who isn't? Come talk to me. I need you."

Then the next call came. "The cancer is in remission, but I've had three small heart attacks, they said, and my MS is flaring up again. Come over and let me fix pancakes for us with tea and we'll talk."

Three weeks later the phone rings. "Are you sitting down? I have three brain tumors. I'm starting radiation. When it's finished I'm going to go to my little part-time job. It helps me to be a little busy like that. The customers see I'm bald and they see my cane and they talk to me. They marvel at my faith and my smile in spite of it all. Come see me."

I called to see how the radiation treatments were going and she said, "You have to come meet my new husband. He is a saint. I want you to come and sit and we'll talk again. I am not afraid to die. And look, I'm still here. See, I'm not done until I'm done! I'm trusting God totally with all of this. If He wants me to stay longer, then I'm all for that. If He's ready for me to come to Heaven, I'll do my best to be brave and agree to that as well."

Her home greeted me like I was entering a cottage in a lovely storybook. Artwork was everywhere, flowing shawls and porcelain antique tea cups, warm paint colors that graced the furniture, the books and the lighting from little decorative lamps. And she was dressed with bright colors, jewelry, soft darling head wraps, and red lipstick.

I held her close and she said, "It's okay. It's really okay. Today we do today. And we trust tomorrow will be what tomorrow needs to be."

"Do you want sugar in your tea?

"Now sit. I want to ask you to be with me when I begin my dying stage."

I was.

CHAPTER 14

RINGTAIL TOOTER

The ambulance crew wheeled Sarah into our treatment room and carefully moved her from the carrier to one of the beds.

"Ohhh, watch it, Sonny. I'm sore from that ride from hell in that contraption you call an ambulance. Gentle there; I'm sure I'm bruised. How'd you get this job? What'd you do with my pink satin pillow? Don't touch my house shoes or I'll clobber ya. Oh, where am I? How long are ya gonna leave me here? Oh, Lord, I bet there's pain involved!" she groaned in high-pitched moans.

She was with us to receive two units of blood, which would take about four to five hours. I started summoning courage as the ambulance "boys" walked away grinning at me with "Have a nice day!"

I sat down beside her and started on some paperwork while the blood was being retrieved from the blood bank downstairs. I reminded her why she was with us and introduced myself, then fluffed her pink pillow and held up her house shoes so she could see them again.

"Now listen, Honey," she began, "I'm eighty-seven years old, and I've never really been sick much at all in my life until this abnormal anemia cropped up. Well, except for the flu in 1918—had it in the war camp when I went to see my first husband. He wasn't worth dying over, so I lived. The second one wasn't either, but the third one was okay. We were married for forty years. But never mind that.

"What I want to say is that I don't want any unnecessary pain. You get one chance to put in that IV needle and, if you don't get it right, you go get the best nurse on the floor. I've been poked enough.

"Hey, where's my house shoes? Oh, here they are.

"And another thing: don't give me AIDS. I have to keep an eye on my house shoes because I was in one of these places once and they stole me blind.

"Did I tell you that I still have my own teeth? Good thing or they'd took them too. It's a cruel world out there. I'd rather be gone. Well, not today. Don't take that as permission to be sloppy with your work!"

I was taping her IV line in place and starting the blood when I noticed that she had stopped talking. I glanced down at her.

"Hey, Honey, this isn't the real me. The real me is nicer. She's down in here," she said while pointing to her chest. "The real me gets quieter sometimes while the scared me rants and raves, trying to sound brave or in control. I used to sell cosmetics years ago... did it for thirty-eight years. Wish you could've known me then. I smelled better, too.

"I just didn't think I'd ever let anything make me old in my mind. Mostly I've been pretty positive, but I know a chronic illness can sneak up on ya with a bad attitude some days. I'm weak when I'm low on blood and I can't seem to muster up the fight as well. I'm tired.

"You nurses probably don't realize how good it is to be so healthy and strong and have all that energy you need to take care of people like me. Did you ever think when it's time to get up in the morning that it's a gift you don't have to wait for someone to come get you up? Put your arm up against mine. I'm all purple blotched and shriveled. No cold cream can fix this. You better appreciate your skin.

36

"Okay, okay, I've gone on enough. By the time we're finished here I'll be feeling better. Go find me some peanut butter and crackers and a Pepsi-Cola...and hurry."

One of the other nurses in the med room stopped me and asked, "Hey, you want me to help you out with her? I hear she can be a ring-tailed tooter!"

"No thanks. I like the ole' gal. I think she's got a story or two to tell me before she goes to sleep, and I bet they're worth hearing."

CHAPTER 15

SAME PERSON

About six forty-five a.m. Larry was the first patient to arrive and unload out of a creaking, outdated elevator. He was here for lab work and outpatient chemotherapy. He approached the reception desk to sign in and let me know he had already been to the laboratory. So now he was waiting on the results to see if they were good enough for him to get this next dose of chemo.

"Good morning!" I said while glancing at the patient sheet for the day, hoping to catch his name without it being so obvious that I had no idea what it was. I was still learning, getting familiar with everyone, staff and patients.

He pointed to his hearing aids and replied, "Even though I have these things, I can't hear much at all. I'm really deaf except for loud noises, but I do lip-read a little."

"Would you like some coffee?" I awkwardly asked, not intending to talk too loudly or too fast or too slowly.

"Yes, please," he answered, smiling at me and appearing to recognize a familiar uneasiness and my attempt to communicate.

He followed me into the waiting room. As I did the morning

38

"chores," he shared with me bits and pieces about himself.

"You know, I've been coming here for treatments for over five years. Now I just come for check-ups and occasionally some chemo. It's a blood cancer is what it is. When they first figured out what I had wrong I was really angry for a while.

Then one evening about dusk while I was putting a milk cow back in the barn with her baby, I thought out loud to myself, "I am the same person I was before this cancer. I can choose to keep living and doing the things I like to do, and who knows how long I have any way! Being angry isn't making me feel any better."

"I think my visits here helped me to see other people worse off than me and it made me decide to choose to just try to live more in my present day and quit worrin' about a tomorrow that hasn't arrived yet. It sure made a difference in how I started sleeping at night.

"That little calf doesn't worry whether or not he's going to grow up to be a champion blue ribbon bull some day. My little terrier trusts that he'll get a ride in my pickup with me to town and doesn't seem to stew about if there's enough dog food in the house.

"I don't feel like I have to tell my grown children how to live their lives anymore either. They'll figure it out one way or another. That's their education. Course now, if they ask me...well I might give them a little advice." He smiled and raised his eyebrows.

"You probably noticed this right hand of mine," he continued. "It's been drawing up like this for years. But the left one's fine. I can't let any of these physical limitations pull me down.

"Now, I understand it's normal to be blue sometimes, but you can't stay sad or it'll suck the life right out of you. The good Lord is worthy of trusting, even if I don't understand. Uh-oh, here comes Nadine. Think I'll try to coax a smile out of her while we're waiting on those blood results."

Off he went with his coffee and greeted Nadine, making her smile within minutes.

I wasn't sure if he was telling me all of that for my education or for his reminder to keep up his down-home variation of "one day at a time." Either way, I heard him and, if my memory doesn't fail me in the future, I hope to pull it out of my brain's files when and if it's needed.

CHAPTER 16

NOT GONNA DO IT!

One evening at the beginning of my shift, I went to see one of my patients, Bertha, to introduce myself.

There she sat in the middle of her bed with her curly black wig half-cocked, showing kinky white tiny hairs peeking out as if they were trying to escape. She had pulled her white circulation hose down around her ankles and she was situating her glasses just in the "right place" on her nose to read her Bible.

"Well, get on in here and help me get this rolling table to quit rolling so I can read without getting sea sick," she said as she greeted me.

Then she pulled her wig off and threw it over to the visitor's chair in the corner and began seriously scratching her mostly bald head.

"I ain't wearing that silly sight of a wig anymore. I never did like those things. It ain't right wearing someone else's hair. If folk don't like my head like this, that's their problem. And another thing, missy, you tell that doctor to get in here so I can talk to him about that transfusion he's a wantin' me to have today.

"Not gonna do it! Period. And that's the word with the bark on it!

41

I'm done getting more blood. It's not doing me any good anymore. What wrong with people in not understanding that when it's time to go, it's time to go? Don't hold on to me with any more tricks of yer trade, missy! And don't you get that wide-eyed look with me! You know, I know what I'm talkin' about!

"What have we come to in this world that we think we need to put someone up in a hospital and force 'em to eat when they ain't hungry no more from their dying process? What do they mean trying to force anyone to drink that nasty white drink with vitamins stirred up in it? Done—I'm done is what, I am!

"Okay, missy, not your fault. You jest got here and you jest the first one I've seen step inside my room since I decided to speak my mind. Sit here a spell in that plastic-coated chair in the corner. Now hear me.

"You know my God loves me and gave me this time here on this sweet and troubled Earth with purpose and an allotted time. I trust Him, child. I believe He knows what He is doing even when I don't.

"I believe we are all born with this knowledge, and we forget it when life gets hard or someone tries to make the world believe He up and died. Sakes alive! He ain't dead just because we know misery here. This world always known misery. It ain't Heaven.

"I want you to know right here and now that I trust His timing with me and I believe without a doubt He is coming for me soon, no matter how long my kids want me to remain, no matter how much medicine they give me, or blood in those bags.

"And that's okay. And you can put that in your paperwork that I said so. This world ain't home. Now I'm repeatin' myself! This place is learning ground where we suffer and we love and we tend to one another's sorrow and wounds. We're here to bless, not curse. We're here to share and not pile up belongings in the storehouse when others is sufferin' without.

"Good Lord Almighty, I've gone to preachin'. Listen, missy, God's callin'. I'm anxious to go home to see my sweet Jesus. I'm seein' my brothers and sisters in my dreams and they all smilin' and wavin'.

42

And that music comes to me they tell about. Go on. Get outta here and tell that doctor 'fore they bring up another bag of someone's blood that another soul needs besides me. Tell that doctor what I say."

Then she pulled me close to her giant bosom and hugged me hard and patted my head.

She was done talking.

CHAPTER 17

BODY LANGUAGE

With unmistakable reluctance, Elaine approached our department's reception desk for outpatient oncology, signed her name and, with continued hesitation, quietly entered our waiting room, and sought out a deserted corner to be seated.

She looked more like a model for *Vogue* than a patient in treatment. She was six feet tall, slender, very well dressed, as in pink cashmere suit with stylish leather shoes and bag to match, sculptured nails, a glowing complexion, and soft, wavy chestnut brown hair that brushed her shoulders as she entered.

But demanding attention above all else was the body language that screamed, "I DO NOT want to be here."

As she seated herself in the chair by my desk and removed her jacket and rolled up her silk sleeve of her blouse she turned her head the other way. I got her vital signs. Then as bravely as I could I asked her, "Is there anything I can get for you while you wait to see the doctor?"

With lowered eyes and trembling hands, she began: "I'm here to have my lab work done. I had chemo last week in the hospital after a recurrence was discovered with my previous week's check-up. My hair will start falling out soon. You know it took me several months to get this length back. You see, I've already done all this before. I'm not ready to face it again."

I sat down, trying not to disturb her outpouring. It did not matter who I was. I just happened to be there when she decided to release, to vent, to verbally resent an unwelcomed return of her cancer. All she wanted from me was to be still and listen.

"It's not so much the thought of me losing my hair again," she continued, "it's more that I thought we were past this part. I didn't plan on it coming back. I don't want to read the articles describing different ways to tie a head scarf or wear a cute hat or fix a wig to look like my hair use to."

Her arms were tightly folded across her chest. She was balanced on the edge of her cold metal chair with her long legs crossed, nervously shaking one foot.

"My family is supportive. I know I am loved, and I realize there are probably some here who have no one." She spoke as if voicing a positive blessing was necessary before she continued.

"But...?" I asked, sensing there was much more.

"But, I am not even sure if I want to do this again. Do you understand?" she asked, following her painful confession.

I hesitated and then answered, "Honestly, no. I cannot say I understand any of what you feel because I have not been where you are. I have not been faced with your decision. You alone know what is right for you. Regardless, whatever you decide we will respect that choice. Either way, we are here for you."

Then she started crying. "I know," she whispered while blotting her mascara-stained tears.

Then she walked over to an elderly woman who was bald and weak and smiling and said, "Can I sit by you? Would you like a cup of coffee or tea while we wait?"

Years before, when I worked on the oncology unit in the hospital, I was shocked when I first heard a patient say that they didn't want any more chemo.

In that break room I approached the supervisor and said, "Doesn't he know that his family is counting on him to continue? Can't we do something to convince him to change his mind?"

She invited me to follow her to her office.

"We are not here to judge anyone's decision. How do you know that he is making the wrong choice? We are here to follow doctors' orders, educate, keep the patients safe, answer their questions, listen to them, and keep them as comfortable as possible. We allow each person their right to decide if and how they proceed with their options."

"And," she continued while placing a hand on my shoulder, "if you can carry that into your personal life as well, it'll save you a lot of grief."

CHAPTER 18

NEIGHBORLY HOUSEKEEPING

While working one evening on the oncology floor I noticed Mr. Jones, an elderly gentleman who was curled into a fetal position on his bed, lying motionless for what seemed like a long time.

I tiptoed closer to see if he was awake. As his peripheral vision caught my movement, he looked up through his inch-thick glasses with black rims.

"Hello, Mr. Jones. I thought I'd drop by and see about you before I start an IV on your neighbor around the corner." I smiled while inching closer to his good ear.

"Oh," he said, "well, have a seat next to me on this thing they call a bed and I'll tell you a couple of things I've been waiting to say to whoever my evening nurse might be. If you're wondering, like the morning nurse, about how much I'm eating...I'm not. A feller can force that institutional food down only so long.

"And, if they come in here again to stick me for some foreign blood test, they'd better get ready fer a fight!" he continued. "There's no such thing as sleep day or night in this joint. Someone wakes me up at four in the morning to weigh me! Who the hell thought that was a good idea?"

"Now, course I'll do as the doc says, but, well, reckon I'm just tired."

He turned to look at me, I think for a reaction.

"Well, we'll see if we can get your weight at another time that's more suitable. Maybe I can get the nutritionist to come talk to you about options for your diet. But you will have to take it up with your doc about those 'foreign' blood tests."

"Oh, it's all right, sister. I know I signed on for all this when I told the doctor I wanted to fight this. But do you know what? There is some good news. Some lady came in here a while ago and made this bed and set down with me and watched television. Wasn't that nice of her? She didn't even know me."

I glanced around his room as he spoke and noticed how bare it was. No cards, no flowers, no fancy robe or leather slippers, no sign of a family or a friend. No one, nothing.

"Yes, yes, it was very nice of her," I answered.

"Well, I'll check on you again after dinner and see if you were able to get a better tray. I have to start that IV next door. You push that nurse button if you need us."

As I pulled his door to almost shut, I thought to myself, "He didn't even realize that the nice lady was from housekeeping."

I wondered if she had any idea how much pleasure she had brought the man in Room 102 just by tuning in her favorite soap opera while making his bed.

What power we possess with a moment or two—a simple smile, an affirmative tip of the hat, a single rose, holding a car door open. The list is endless.

CHAPTER 19

I'LL SEE YA WHEN I SEE YA

Jane's sister-in-law, Sue, carried Jane's black patent purse and lightly quilted jacket, following closely behind her, just in case Jane lost her balance while Jane carried her trusty walker more than using it for its intended purpose. The sister-in-law spoke first.

"She's real grouchy today, Becki. Better watch her. She's almost mean!"

They both grinned. But from the looks of her facial expressions and body language, I wasn't sure it was a joking matter.

"Don't worry about me. I'm not scared of her. Why I'm about as ornery. Who wants coffee?" I teased back at them.

"Coffee?! You call that coffee?!" My walker-toting gal came back.

"Who'd want that? Tastes more like medicine to me. Hey, by the way, those scales in the reception room aren't accurate. I don't weigh that much. And another thing: it's cold as an icebox in here. Don't you guys pay your heating bill?"

"Come on, let's get you in a blanket and put you in an exam room before you frighten someone," I continued in jest.

But, alone in the room and away from the crowd, a serious face replaced the tired smile. Catching me off guard, she asked. "You got any answers?"

"To which questions?" I quizzed in return, not sure yet of the direction she was heading.

"Well, I don't rightly know. There's so many. How's a person supposed to pay these kind of medical bills when they're too weak to work? How does anyone make any sense out of those insurance forms? How do you eat when you've lost so much weight your dentures slide around and your appetite has flat-out disappeared...like it all taste like chewed-up rubber bands or cardboard? How do you find the desire to take a walk to build up your strength when you're afraid of a draft or a flu bug germ hiding around the corner? How do I switch from my independent life to one of people hovering over me? How do I cope with what I'm uncertain about? And....how long?"

I put aside my supplies.

"Now, nurse, I don't expect you to have an answer for every one of my questions. But I can't say this stuff at home. My sister-in-law—God love her—folds like a cheap lawn chair when I get serious and ask her a question about death. Most folks don't do too well with getting uneasy about things I want to ask. So I saved it up for you. I know you people up here in this clinic have connections. I need some answers even if I don't like 'em. Okay, now I'm done talking. Do your deal then; go get me some of that nasty coffee." She finished with a weak smile.

I talked to her doctor and my supervisor, and they visited with her before we began her chemo preparations, making connections with dietary, hospice, insurance liaisons, etc., who all said they would visit briefly with her and make appointments to come to her home to visit more or call her.

Her doctor talked to her about her treatments and her prognosis.

I headed to the pharmacy to pick up her chemo. The girl at the window there said, "The doctor just phoned us and said Ms. Jones has decided not to take any more chemo. He said she just needs a break and he's not going to argue with her today."

As I was getting off the elevator back to our clinic, here she came with a broader smile now.

"Hey, nurse, I'll see ya when I see ya!" she winked and carried her walker into the elevator.

I don't think the doctor realized yet that she wouldn't be making an appointment for him to try to "argue with her."

CHAPTER 20

BEING GOOD STEWARDS

Some who came for outpatient chemo were shy and hid behind a book or a magazine with an imaginary sign that said, "Do not disturb!"

Some weren't.

But every Wednesday morning when I arrived at the clinic, John was already there. No one would have ever guessed he was dealing with a terminal diagnosis and prognosis. Without a shy bone in his body he would cheerfully "Howdy!" everyone as they came in for treatment or blood work.

He would question each patient about their well-being and enjoyed kidding around with anyone who felt up to it.

I never once heard him quote scripture or recite a sermon, but I sensed this elderly gentleman was intimately acquainted with his God.

"Please now, sister, don't put me in one of those exam rooms until the doctor gets here. I'd rather sit out here in the waiting room and visit a while," he requested of me. "Sure, John, I'll come back and get you when it's your turn," I replied.

From a distance, I would watch him with the pride and pleasure of seeing him "work the room."

Some days the entire wait was spent with only one other patient. During other visits, he would make it around the room, checking on as many as possible before his turn.

One evening, a few weeks later, he was admitted to the hospital in-patient wing. When I found out he was in the hospital I hurried up to see him after all our patients were finished with their treatments. I peered around the door to his private room, and he turned and reached for me with both arms open wide.

"Sister, sister, come in here. Sweet of you to be here. How is everyone in the outpatient clinic?"

"We're all fine, John. How about you?" I asked as I moved a chair close to his bedside.

"Well, Honey, I guess the ole' rascal is growing again. We'll have to fight harder. I'll not give up today."

As I looked up from his determined expression, I saw the room was full of colorful posters and cards with get well wishes all over the walls, the bathroom door, and the windows:

"Get well, Pops!" and "We love you, Pops!"

There were signatures from Sunday school classes, youth groups, prayer groups, family, neighbors, and community leaders.

I drew in a big breath of courage and spoke while taking his hands in mine, "John, I want you to know how pleased I am to know you. I watch you each week in the waiting room, and I sense from these posters and cards that the nice way you treat everyone is part of your normal routine. The regular patients have been asking about you. They miss your comments. You know, your talent is special."

Tears rolled down his fevered, blushed cheeks.

"We must sow seeds for the Master while we have the chance and trust another to water them, and another to reap," he said. "We are to be good stewards of our time here, sister."

They moved John to ICU the next day.

After lunch I ran up the stairs for a visit.

53

"Could you please tell me which room John is in?" I asked the nurse at the desk while catching my breath.

With a lowered voice she answered, "They moved him about thirty minutes ago to the morgue. The funeral home from his community is on the way. I'm so sorry. Did you know him as a patient or as a friend?"

"Both."

CHAPTER 21

THE COWBOY AND CHEMO

One of the best bits of wisdom shared by more than one of my patients over the years was a question posed to me like this: "What kind of footprints do you want to leave behind on this Earth?"

I was working the Oncology Outpatient Clinic in Tulsa at the time I first heard those words. Samuel was in a brown faux leather recliner with his swollen feet propped up while I was studying his compromised veins for one suitable enough to start an IV that would carry the caustic chemo to him safely.

He was quieter than usual and seemed to me to be "dealing" with something that day, more than where he was going to go after his chemo. He rarely had any nausea afterward and wanted to go out to eat while in the "big city."

I found the precious vein and got the IV going. I put on my gown and gloves, started the pre-meds, and was arranging my little bedside table with his chemo, tape, and a syringe when he spoke.

"Becki, what kind of footprints do you want to leave behind on this Earth?"

"Huh?" I looked up a little surprised and asked.

"Well, I been thinking. Just in case this doesn't come out okay, and I might be headin' out of here sooner than later, I was wonderin' what I might be remembered for while I've been on this ole' Earth.

"The only words my neighbor on the west end of the farm hears from me is me cussing those cows on a regular basis. My wife's mother sees me leave the room right quick when she comes over for another visit. My kids seldom hear a word out of me less it's aggravating them about stuff like, 'Did you do your homework? Did you feed those steers? Did you close that gate? Did you help your mother with getting that feed sack out of the trunk of the car?' And all I ever do in church is walk in, sit in the back pew, give them a couple of dollars, and leave before the preacher quits saying his final prayer. Nice guy, but he sure likes to hear himself talk!"

"Why Samuel, you've always been very nice to all of us up here," I said. "I can't imagine you've left too many bad footprints." I patted his other hand.

"Oh, shucks, who's gonna be rude to you girls! You have the needles!" he said with a huge grin.

"Okay then, Samuel, what would you do different?" I asked while slowly infusing the medications.

"Well, that's what I've been dwelling on here lately. I'm not a religious sort of fella by any means, but I do like God. I think God is okay. I've just never been too fond of some church folk and some ministers. They aren't all bad, but some of 'em talk outta both sides of their mouths!

"But now I'm rethinking it a little. Church isn't for perfect people. There aren't any! Church is for all of us! I might cuss and the other fellow might be a snob. We BOTH can sit in that pew. I'm going to work on not judging them anymore and I'm going to give them a five-dollar bill instead of two dollars. And I'm going to let him shake my hand before I run out that door.

"And I've decided I'm going to quit yelling at my kids. I want

56

them to have some good memories. I'm going to make an effort to sit down with all the family at dinner instead of eating in front of that TV with my old Roy Rogers TV tray. They're good kids. And I couldn't have a better wife. I need to tell her that, I reckon.

"Now it might take me a few days to improve on hanging out with my mother-in-law some more, but she too means well. She's not a really bad sort.

"And I think I'm going to drive the pick-up truck over to the neighbor's house and tell him how much I appreciate him chopping that ice on the pond for my cows a few weeks ago when the kids were in school and my wife was at work. I didn't have the energy to swing an axe. He just got out there and did that for me and never said a word. I hope I'd have done the same for him.

"Another reason I started in thinking about all this was because we went to a funeral the other day and there was standing room only in that little church house.

"I can tell you right here and now that our friend was making the finest footprints here on Earth you've ever heard tell of. Not a soul didn't like him and respect him. There's never been a doubt about how he felt about his God and his family and his community. And same goes for his church and his neighbors. He had a dairy farm, wasn't wealthy by any means, worked from sun up to sun down and still took the time to share what he had with others, whether it was milk or green beans or corn or okra or tomatoes. You should have heard the testimonies given at that service. His preacher hardly had a chance to preach due to so many needing to say what this man meant to them.

"I was sitting there on that back pew in that service embarrassed to think, *Who'd stand up for me?*

"I just sat there after finishing the chemo and glanced around the room. Not a dry eye was to be seen. The four other patients in recliners and their family members were blotting their eyes with Kleenex.

I pulled him up close and whispered, "Do you know what you

57

have done for so many today with this visit? You have preached one of the finest sermons anyone of us has ever heard! You, my dear friend, have left GOLDEN footprints here today."

He quietly got up after I put a band aide on his IV site. He put on his sweat-stained cowboy hat, politely nodded at all those he passed, and went to the elevator.

PART TWO
HOSPICE GIFTS

CHAPTER 1

DO YOU SEE THEM?

When I was working for the big city hospital's brand new hospice I was visiting the cutest little Pentecostal minister you've ever seen. He had a shock of white hair and bright, baby blue eyes. He lived next door to his church built in the '50s and was surrounded with ancient oaks. He lived with his second wife, Matilda. She called him "the Reverend Smith" since she was one of his parishioners before his first wife died. She thought it was disrespectful to call him by his first name.

Matilda liked to stay in the kitchen when I came to visit, but I tried to get her to listen to all I was saying to her husband about hospice. She would flap her flowered full-bodice apron, turn on her heels, and run off again.

One day while sitting at my desk at work the receptionist, leaned around my cubicle and said, "Hey, Florence [that's what she called all the nurses], that lady that calls and screams about her husband needing help just called and said to hurry on over there."

I called her to reassure her that I was on my way and tried to repeat the info we had gone over. I told her to call her next door neighbor and see if she would come and be with them till I got there.

When I arrived my sweet patient was sitting straight up in his trusty rocking recliner struggling for air with a serious color of blue taking over his face. "Can you get me to my bed? I want to see out that picture window."

I picked him up and carried him to his quilt-covered bed and straddled him, holding him up as straight as I could so he could breathe better. Matilda ran back into the kitchen with her face in her apron and the neighbor ran home.

Dear Brother Smith patted my fingers on his left shoulder. "Do you see them?" he gasped with excitement.

"No, sir, but tell me. What are you seeing?" I whispered back into his ear.

"The room here is now full of angels. 'Tilda, come quick. I've got to go now. I'll see you again, Honey...later on." He tried to comfort her.

Off she went again to her safety net.

He lifted up his right hand into the air and called out, "My Lord. My Lord and my God." And then he fell back against me with his last breath.

I just sat there for several minutes until Tilda came back into the living room, surprisingly, calm now. She helped me lay his head down on his feather pillow and I held her a while. She didn't run away anymore.

Some say it's a lack of oxygen, some say it's due to pain medication or organ failure. Me? I'm proud I got to be there.

CHAPTER 2

DOES GOD LOVE ME?

Donnie wasn't quite thirty years old. He had come back to Oklahoma to be with his mom while he was dying. Cancer was the written diagnosis on the assignment sheet. But in reality, it was AIDS; it was the 1980s.

"Don't tell anyone what my real diagnosis is, please. I'm afraid they will torment my mother after I'm gone," he pleaded.

Being so very tall, he barely fit on the hospital bed we had delivered. He had me put on all the advised protection to give him his bed bath or shave him or empty his catheter bag. I had on booties, gown, gloves, and mask. As awful as it all was, we would laugh at how I looked.

One morning as I was gently as possible cleaning his open wounds, he whispered, "Becki, does God love me?"

I looked up and said, "Yes, Donnie, God loves you. God loves me. God loves every one of us."

"But will you have a minister come talk to me?" he asked.

"Yes, we'll have one come today if you'd like."

My supervisor called this most amazing minister who came and spent time with Donnie; the minister talked to him, prayed with him, and reassured him of God's love for him while I stood in the living room with his exhausted mother, who wept until her eyes were nearly swollen shut.

As the weeks progressed, he wasn't able to speak anymore but would look at me with his beautiful blue eyes expressing gratitude. I would hold his hand and pat his shoulder and whisper up close. "Yes, Donnie. God loves you, God loves me, and God loves everyone."

Bless that minister's heart.

CHAPTER 3

WHO'S IN CHARGE?

Leonard warned me the day I was making my first hospice visit with him and his wife, "Today is the only day you get to talk about this stuff. I'll answer all your questions and you can answer any I have, but then we won't discuss my disease or my prognosis again. You just come and check my vital signs and help me with my pain and teach my wife what she needs to know and that's that. Okay?"

"Yes, sir. We will do this your way."

So that's exactly how we handled our visits. We would talk about the cows in the pasture and the chickens in the chicken house or the coon dog out in the fenced-in area they had fixed up for him so he wouldn't chase the cows or the eat the chickens. And every now and then we would talk about the weather, but he didn't want to talk forecast, just weather for that day.

One day he said, "Listen, you've been right nice about adhering to my wishes. I thank you. But, you see, today is the day I'm concerned about. Just the right now right here at hand. I don't see any need discussin' what's not here yet. We all know I'm terminal.

Who the hell isn't? Think about that for a minute. I think we have to line things out best we can as we know about them and then just do what chore lies before us. That's all I got to say about that today. You might need to spend more time with my wife anyway."

I went into the kitchen and sat at the little aluminum table with Betty and asked her if I could do anything for her before I left. "Well, what would that be? Let's see, I heard tell you ain't got much of a gift for cooking. And I heard you're not too hot with cross-stitching or canning green beans or milking cows. What did you have in mind? You got anything in that nurse's bag of yours to make any of this any better?"

"No, I guess not. But I'm good at laundry," I said as I looked down at the kitchen's linoleum floor.

At that point she chuckled. "Well, shoot fire! Let's fold some laundry."

That's what we did for an hour or so while she unloaded some verbal pain about how hard it was to try to honor his wishes not to talk about what was staring her in the face. She wanted to talk to the funeral home but he did not. She wanted him to talk to their sons. He did not. So she continued to talk to us nurses or her sister. She said she even took to talking to the coon hound every now and then, and he seemed to understand as well as anyone.

CHAPTER 4

FACE TO FACE WITH ANGER

In the early 1990s I was visiting hospice patients all over northeast Oklahoma. My supervisor called me into her office and sat me down. "I want you to go see a fellow who's dying with lung cancer."

"And...?" I asked with suspicion. She usually just gave me the assignments.

"Well, it's not your everyday death and dying case. He's angry. Just don't take it personal," she added as she dismissed me.

So far I hadn't had an "everyday death and dying case."

Tom and his wife lived in a mobile home in a rural setting. A pack of dogs, kind of like the "Bumpus Hounds" in the *Christmas Story* movie, met me in the front yard by a lean-to porch. They looked neglected, but that can happen if you have to focus 24/7 on taking care of someone.

His wife met me at the door and took me into the kitchen. The info I got said they were in their forties. She looked sixty at least, as thin as a rail, big ole' bags under her eyes, and mousey brown thin hair that didn't look like it had seen shampoo in a while and was pulled back tightly with a green newspaper rubber band.

"That other nurse lady told me over the phone you were coming and I want to talk to you first before you go in there to see Tom," she whispered while wringing her hands.

"You see, he's not in a very good mood, and I'm sorry about that. I hope you won't be scared of him. He used to be nice. But he's real mad about dying. He can't hurt you or anything like that, it's just... well, he's hateful to all of us," she continued with tears running down her face, pooling into the deep space between her collar bones.

"Thank you for that warning. I'll be okay. Anger is not uncommon. I won't take it personal," I said with pride in my knowledge and experience, and without a real clue about what I was getting into. Let me just say that occasionally you walk into stuff that hasn't been written in any nursing book or spoken about in any classroom.

Tom was halfway propped up in the hospital bed in the living room. I was a bit shocked. How on earth could this man still be alive? Dry, yellowing skin pulled tightly over bones, he stood over six feet tall and had dull eyes that once had been blue, his wife had told me.

On each side of the bed were his two sisters. They were whispering to each other and Tom when I approached them. I introduced myself and explained what his doctor had asked us to do for him and his family. He cut his eyes my direction.

"I don't give a shit what the doctor said. What in the hell difference does it make? I'm dying. Doesn't matter what my blood pressure is anymore. My sisters can give me my pain medicine. And I'm not interested in any damn preacher coming by here either to talk to me about God."

He pulled himself up closer to me holding onto the bed rail. "I suppose you talked to my wife. Well, let's set the facts straight. Write this down on your papers. She can't wait till I die. She's been having an affair for quite some time, and they're just biding their time till the undertaker pulls up in the driveway. Why don't you give that report to your boss and my doctor? Now get the hell outta here.

Leave me in peace with my sisters to die."

His poor sisters were weeping and trying to console him and get him comfortable again. I was tripping over my feet, clutching my bag and paperwork when his wife grabbed my elbow and pulled me back into the kitchen.

"I'm so sorry. He's out of his mind. There is no other man. There never has been. He's breaking all our hearts with this. He's so convinced. His doctor told me that his brain has cancer now, too, and his body's organs are beginning to shut down and all his numbers are outta whack and he's just so confused. No matter what we say he doesn't believe us. I never expected this. I was prepared for his dying, I thought, but clearly I'm not."

When he has had his pain meds and he is sound asleep, I go in there, hold his hand, stroke his forehead for a while, and pray. It's all I know to do.

"I thank you for coming and tell your supervisor we'll be okay. I don't think it's going to work out with any more strange people coming in the house. The other day he thought the guy who was delivering propane was suspicious," she said while leading me out onto the porch.

I stopped to put my bag and papers down and then took her bony frame into my arms. I held her and whispered, "I'm so sorry."

I let her cry until she seemed out of tears.

I drove back to the hospital, went right into the supervisor's office, and shut the door.

She looked me over and with a sigh began, "Okay, I told you, remember?

"I want you to listen to what an experienced nurse told me when we took care of dying people in ICU instead of their homes, when I had a similar experience as you did today.

"She said, 'Betty, you need to understand that these end-of-life situations are something like a play. The main and most important character is the patient. The rest of us are supporting actors. This is their story, and this is their final scene. And the success of this is

69

not dependent upon how smart you are or how nice you are or how white and starched your lab coat is. Don't let your ego keep you from being a good nurse.

"'Yes, play your part well. Stay focused on providing the information needed, the comfort (best you can), and emotional support, but back away from center stage. You are not the hero. And there's not a competition for best nurse in here either. It's teamwork. Where you're weak, another is strong, and vice versa. Does no one any good if someone's trying to be some sort of Florence Nightingale. Keep your heart in there, but when it's time to go home, your part's been played. Trust in the other actors to do their job well. There'll be another play tomorrow, another final act.'"

I still think those kind of tidbits of information should be in textbooks or lectures, but I guess you learn it best long after graduation.

One patient once told me, "It's all an education, Becki—ever' bit of life."

CHAPTER 5

HOW THE COW EATS THE CABBAGE OR ELSE

One day I got to go to see a lovely lady in town whose name was Mary Catherine. What a darling house! It had white clapboard siding with pinkish red shutters and a porch swing on the west side of the porch. There were flowers lining the stepping stone walkway to the antique front door. It had an oval beveled glass front and was painted just a shade lighter than the shutters. A late spring breeze carried the scent of peonies to my senses and made me smile all over. Visions of Grandma's flowerbed jumped forward to my thoughts. Then I heard her, "Come on in, door's unlatched."

Oh! The inside was as charming as the outside. There was flowered wallpaper from the '40s on the walls and a china cabinet with pink, cranberry, and green Depression-era glass. There she sat in her overstuffed winged back chair that also had a flowered print on it. She had just the prettiest white hair all pulled back and up, and she was wearing a flannel rose-colored gown with a ruffled apron with maroon rickrack on the top of it. She was holding her TV remote in the pocket on one side and the panic alert button for help in the other pocket.

"Well, come on in, nurse. As you can see, I'm surrounded with all these dishes and antiques, and I'm sorting out what goes to which child and grandchild and niece or nephew. I've got a friend who is going to come over after a bit and put them in their designated boxes. You'd think that this would depress me terribly bad, but it's been a good morning. I'm enjoying looking over each piece and remembering when I got it and what was going on when me and Henry bought it. Bless him. He's been gone nearly twenty-five years now.

"I know you come to check my vital signs and see how my ticker's doing. But, before you do anything else, I want you to sit on that embroidered footstool—not that leather one, it's wobbly—and let me inform you about how the cow eats the cabbage.

"I've been up there in that big city hospital for several days and about a month ago before that. You see my heart is wearing out. I've died twice and they shocked the snot out of me and brought me back both times. I've told them as plain as I could before I left that ICU room that they're not to do that anymore. I was already having the blessing of seeing Heaven and feeling the peace that we don't have here on this realm, when BAM! I'm back in my cold ole' body and feeling all that pain and bother. Lordy!!

"I'm too old for a heart transplant. I don't want any surgery or another pacemaker or another valve replacement. I want to go on. It'll happen again and, when it does, if anyone does that CPR stuff on me and puts me on that breathing machine, I'll haunt them if I do get to die!!"

I listened and wrote everything down. My supervisor had already told me that she didn't want any CPR but that she was home to die. But she needed to spit it out and make sure that everyone knew she meant business.

Her heart was very weak but her spirit was strong, and she worked hard on those belongings. A friend and a neighbor and a niece came to box it up before I left while she was dozing quietly in her chair.

72

We were scheduled to visit again the next day and help her with some laundry and some skin care and I was going to sneak out there and cut some of her flowers to put in a Roseville pottery vase I saw on her kitchen counter. But as I was making out my schedule for the day with my assignments, the call came in from her family. The neighbor found her that morning in her chair. She was gone.

I couldn't help but smile. She and Henry.

CHAPTER 6

THE SWEETEST SOUND

Ryan was eleven years old and was HIV positive in a world that was scared silly about the disease.

"Don't tell anybody, okay, nurse?" he asked with all the seriousness in the world. "I don't want anyone burning my mama's house down just because they are scared they will get AIDS from us. I read about that Florida boy." At such a young age he was aware of much more than many.

But his mother and family decided to do their best to keep him as happy as possible with all he was facing and all the treatments and IVs—the robbery of a childhood.

"He got this from his blood transfusion when we lived in California. There's nothing fair about it, but it is what it is, and we're making the best of it as we can." She told me matter-of-factly.

She was a tiger of a mom and watched out for him 24/7 with a whole bunch of love. He would be watching cartoons while we were infusing medication, and he would call her name over and over, "Mama? Mama? Mama?" and she would come running. "Yes, son? What is it?"

And he would reply, "I was seeing if you were still here. That's all." Then he would go back to his show and she would go back to doing dishes or the laundry.

One day I asked her in private, "Does that make you crazy, with him calling your name over and over several times a day?"

She stopped what she was doing and looked at me, trying not to cry, and said, "That voice is the sweetest sound I've ever heard, and I'm trying to memorize it. What makes me crazy it that one day it will be quiet in here."

"Please forgive me. I'm so sorry."

She went back to doing dishes.

Later I made it a point to tell my friends, "When you are tired of hearing those kiddos scream, stop and thank the good Lord for their dear little voices. Stop and look at their artwork they bring you from school, and tape it up on the refrigerator. Take more pictures and videos, and tell them how special their work is. Read them another bedtime story, and play catch with them one more time."

CHAPTER 7

I'M IN CHARGE OF WHO'S COMING AND GOING

When I went to see her husband, Samuel, the very first time, I was more interested in her than him. What a presence! Marjorie was in charge and there was no denying that. They had been married fifty-plus years, and she had seen him through two strokes and now cancer. They were putting the hospital bed up in the living room where he could look out at the cows in the pasture, see the pond, and watch his dog chase the cat back and forth across the fenced-in yard.

"While these medical equipment boys are in there working on putting that contraption of a bed together, come on into the kitchen where we can do that paperwork. Samuel is resting okay on that couch. He'll be fine until we get this necessary evil done."

She had hair like Katherine Hepburn did in her later years. It was reddish and whitish and curly and wavy, and it was pulled loosely up in a knot of sorts. She was wearing a multi-colored, caftan-like garment that flowed behind her when she walked with her head held high, almost like an entrance that I would have imagined Queen Cleopatra making in front of all those people watching her come into Solomon's empire.

I glanced back at Samuel. He had a faint smile and winked at me.

"What all do you need to know besides all his numbers and our phone number and address? Oh and here is the list of medications he's taking. But, to be honest, I don't think he will take all of them. At this point Sam and I have decided he takes only what he feels will make him more comfortable, and he eats only what he wants to eat with no restrictions. And, if he wants to go out on the porch, well, as long as I'm able with our grandson's help, he's going to get to go out on the porch where it's shaded so he can smell that hay being put up after it's cut Saturday and he can see those dern cows.

"I'm in charge of who is coming and going. There's one fool of a neighbor down east of here who is nothing but nosey, and that's not going to be allowed in here. She just wants to come in here and see what she can see and then go back to the quilting club and gab her lips off about our business. No, sir. Not going to happen.

"But then there are a few neighbors who have their hearts in the right place and they can come as I deem proper as to the time of day and accordin' to how Sam's feeling. One of them likes to bring a pear pie she bakes like an apple pie from her abundance of pears off those trees she's had over forty years. He may eat only one bite but it still tickles her that he does. I think she's had a crush on him for years, and didn't think I'd ever noticed. Silly ole' gal.

"And there's the Amish brothers who'll come with their buggy and bring some yeast rolls and summer sausage and maybe some pickle relish that their wives make every summer. They're awful nice people. Sam likes to talk to them even though they don't say too much.

"His sisters will come in tonight and sit a while. They're useless but they mean well. One can't boil water, but she's nice enough. The other one talks the legs off a milk stool. But here's the thing. Once again, it's what he likes and he loves those two like corncakes. They tire out easy so they won't stay long.

"Don't try to tell me what he needs to eat or drink or how often to make him take some of that pain medicine. I'll give it as he needs it, like the doctor said, and he's never taken advantage of that, so don't worry.

"Don't send anyone out here to pray for us either. We pray together and we appreciate everyone's concern, but we're private people about our religious affairs. We've already talked to our preacher, and he knows how Sam wants his service and he's picked out the songs and he doesn't want anyone getting up there and going on about all the good he's done in this county. He said that's bragging, and he thinks that erases all the good anyone does. I agree.

"I can promise you and his doctor, I'll care for him like nobody's business. It'll be my face he sees as he passes and my hand on his and my lips upon his sweaty brow."

"What else do you need to know?"

"Nothing. I believe you. No one could do this better."

Some people run from death as hard and as fast as they can. Some people cozy up to it, bring all the creature comforts, and say, "Tell me how to sit with you."

CHAPTER 8

SISTERS THROUGH THICK AND THIN

It was a very hot summer day. Sweat was rolling down my back making my uniform stick to me, giving me chills. I was bending over to get supplies out of my trunk to take into sisters Ann and Sue. They were in their eighties but had lived together after both of their husbands passed. Now the younger sister (by two years) had breast cancer. She had just returned from the hospital.

"Hey, nurse! Come on in here when you get ready. I'm leaving this screen door unhooked for ya. I need to answer Sue. She's hollering from her bedroom," she said while waving, pointing, and grinning.

The house was probably less than 1,000 square feet and had a postage-stamp–sized front yard with brittle brown grass poking up like little sticks. Their lilac bush looked like it might not make it to next spring. I feared that no one had time to water the yard or the plants. They were busy with their new reality.

Inside the front door, Kitty Kat greeted me by rubbing up against my legs. I looked down and black cat fur was sticking to my already sweaty legs. But she needed to be petted anyhow. Again, I surmised that she had been neglected as of late.

The spotless but faded linoleum floor creaked a little while I walked back toward the bedroom where Ann was waiting with Sue. "Well, nurse lady, come on in. You can see that sister here has done a fine job of tending to my bandage on this chest where they did that there surgery to whack off my breast."

"Ann! Good Lord! What on earth are you talking like that for? I'm sorry, nurse. She's ornery and, since she came home, her sense of humor has done gone whacko."

They were both grinning and snorting; then they started laughing again after they got to snorting!!

She was right. The dressing change had been done with expert care. The wound was clean and dry, and there were no signs of infection around the staples.

"Are you having any pain?" I asked while taking notes as I was checking her pulse. I looked at her ankles and watched her chest rise and fall.

"Nope, none to speak of really. The doctor gave me some of them there narcotic pills but we hid them in the back bedroom in a shoebox under the bed in case some dope addicts come looking for them," she said. Both sisters nodded in agreement.

"I don't want to get all crazy on that dope like some do. I can just take Tylenol and be fine. Is it okay if we go ahead and flush that dope?"

"Well, you might want to keep it a while longer just in case. I'll ask your doctor about prescribing something not quite as strong to help with the discomfort."

"Oh, hell, Sue, go ahead and tell her. We done flushed it. We just didn't want any trouble. I'm not hurting any—well, not very much anyhow."

Then they got to laughing again and started snorting and giggling.

We finished the assessment and went into the kitchen to have a glass of freshly brewed ice tea. When Sue went outside to take Kitty

Kat some fresh water to her place by the back door, Ann leaned toward me. "Hey, listen, what am I suppose to do about Sue not wanting to talk about me maybe dying one day? She stops me cold in my tracks when I try to tell her how I want things to be just in case. The doctor said this cancer, well...we got to it too late. It's spread to my ribs and a few other spots, and I've chosen not to do any treatments. I'm too old, and I'm ready to go on. But my sister sees different. She thinks I should do everything they offer. She's a little ticked off at me right now. What am I going to do?"

I could see Sue was still out in the back yard getting some towels off the clothesline. I leaned closer to Ann. "I think she just loves you so much that she's just not ready yet to think about all this. Give her some time. Be patient with her resistance. As she allows, keep telling her how you feel, and maybe she'll come around in a few days or weeks."

"It's my body, but I think I'd feel the same way if it were her in my shoes. We been seeing after each other for some time now, and I think she's afraid to be alone again like after Fred died. I think that man down at the church that likes to sit next to us would spend time with her, but she's not too excited about all the silliness that these old men get into when they're wanting you to marry them after one or two dinner dates." She grinned again and winked.

Sue slammed the back screen door. "Well those damn birds done pooped on my white towels!"

Once again both of them are laughing and carrying on.

I left that day not a bit worried about the heat. I was thinking of them and praying the good Lord would keep their humor going, their love for each other strong, and a peace to come in their different ways of thinking.

CHAPTER 9

CAN'T JUDGE BY THE HAIRSTYLE— YOURS OR MINE!

I was asked to go to an Amish community northwest of town one day to visit a family who was caring for their mother who had surgery and now had a stomach tube in her side; she couldn't swallow anymore.

Back in those days, I had bright red short spiky hair. (Well, some days it was orange red and some days it was maroon—even dark brown once or twice.) Also I wore bright red lipstick. My supervisor looked at me with her hands on her hips and sighed, "Well, if we're lucky, maybe they'll notice how kind you are."

When I arrived the living room was full of people. Their mom's bed was situated in the middle of the spotless hardwood living room floor. There wasn't much furniture or extras. There was an oak table covered with a bleached white cloth that had all the necessary equipment to attend to my patient's abdominal wound, care of the tubing, a pole and tubing for the feedings, a large syringe, water in a white porcelain pitcher and the medications prescribed. The smallest of the children who weren't busy doing their chores were anxious to watch me take care of their grandma.

But I couldn't help but notice their eyeballs bug out when I first walked in the house. I don't think they had ever seen anyone as foreign as me. But Sarah was the spokesperson and stepped forward and introduced herself and some of the others. They just nodded.

I went over to introduce myself to my patient as well. She looked up at me and smiled, weakly nodding. She offered one wrinkled, soft, powder white hand to me while the other one didn't move. Sarah shooed the children outside, and the one brother went out as well. The women stepped forward and we began. I praised them for the perfect care they had given this much loved woman. She was freshly bathed and her hair was braided and wrapped around the crown of her head. Her skin had been covered in baby lotion and she smelled like Ivory soap. Her urine catheter was clean and her heels and tail bone showed no signs of breakdown. We reviewed the tube feedings and the care of the insertion site of the tube into her abdominal wall and how to give the medications and measure her intake and output and monitor her discomfort. They could not have been better nurses, they were the best.

With each visit the family became a little more used to me and trusted me. I got a little brave one day and asked them how they kept up with all the chores. One was cooking homemade noodles and chicken just after killing the chicken! Another was canning corn and green beans, and another had come in from driving the tractor across the field for an errand. I told them I would have been fired as an Amish woman if I'd been born there. I thought all chickens needed to keep their necks. I'd burn food in the pots before I'd ever get it to the table. I might be good at driving a tractor, but I'd be resentful if I wasn't able to speak my piece and drive it where I wanted. They all looked at me and started laughing. Thank goodness!!

Their sweet mom passed away suddenly one day with another stroke. I was charting in my little cubicle a couple of weeks after that and I looked up and there stood Sarah. She had come to town with that tractor and a wagon and brought me a huge tray of goodies: whole wheat buns, applesauce, cookies, a pie, fresh bread, and pickles. I was so grateful and humbled. I thanked her. She said, "Thank you for telling us we did a good job with my mom." We can't judge anyone by how they look or what they wear. We can't see their hearts. Jesus said, only God can do that.

When anyone looks at my grandson with his tattoos and big earrings and long hair and make faces, I think, "You have no idea how beautiful his soul is how huge his heart is." I can't judge them for making faces either. Might be they just had gas!

CHAPTER 10

CHAPLAIN OR NURSE

After several years of nursing I wanted to become a hospice chaplain and went to a two-year program with a church and became a lay minister and got to be a hospice chaplain for a while. This was a challenge for me. I would go into a home to visit a patient and see if they needed a different pain med or that there was a new skin ulcer evident on their elbow that needed attention. I would call and tell the supervisor, "Hey, Mable's blood pressure is dropping and her oxygen's low and her sister wants her to have it. I don't think Mable does, but I need to get back in there and pray with her, so will you tell her nurse?" I could see my supervisor's eyes rolling. I was trying not to step on too many toes. Didn't work well.

I loved being able to sit with the patient's caregivers while the nurse was there so I could focus on them. Being the caregiver all day and all night is a big job. But all of a sudden I would go from listening to them share about their fatigue and their heartache and start telling them how important it was that they get a break and ask about their physical status—if they were sleeping okay, if they had taken their blood pressure medication, and if someone had been able to feed the dog that day. After about a year or two (I can't remember for sure), I decided to take a break and look into just being a volunteer.

To this day, I'll go visit someone who has called and I'm eyeballing their skin, asking about how effective their pain med is, how fast they are breathing a minute, if their kidneys are shutting down, and if they would like a prayer while looking at the cat's dish.

I can see it all now. I'll be in some nursing home in Sedona, Arizona, or Florida with John in one recliner and me in the other. I'll be up trying to check his pulse and he'll think I'm the lady next door and wink at me and say, "Hey, I think my wife's asleep, want to smooch?"

And then I'll fall over laughing so hard I won't be able to catch my breath good and I'll die in his recliner instead of mine.

Old habits die hard, I don't care who you are.

CHAPTER 11

GOOD LUCK?

The doctor that called asking us to go see his dying patient at her home had waited until right up to the end to call.

"She hasn't wanted to bother anyone with anything and felt like they could handle everything from their end, but her pain is worse and she can't swallow very well. I'd like for you to give her some IV morphine with the smallest needle you have. Her veins are nearly gone. And good luck."

"Good luck?! Good luck?!" I was thinking while driving to the house. Three daughters were standing in the doorway and a brother or two in the living room waiting on me.

"Oh, thank goodness you're here. We can't get her pills down her anymore and we are so anxious to get her some pain relief. Can you help us?" they asked as all three of them seemed to move in unison with me toward her bedroom.

It was a tiny bedroom but one that had all the kids' senior class photos on the wall and figurines that looked like Hummels that meant a lot to her, and a chenille bedspread in white, pink, and baby blue. So it was more than evident they had been trying to make her as comfortable as possible.

I couldn't believe she was still among the living. She was so dehydrated and tiny, almost like a bird with some human spirit inside. She looked up at me and weakly smiled.

I told her that her doctor had called us and requested that we help her with some pain medication and that I would try very carefully to get the teeny tiny needle in her teeny tiny vein to deliver some relief. She nodded with agreement and permission.

All the children scurried out of the room for fear of their mom being hurt in the process. They wanted her to know pain relief, not increased pain. And I was praying like you know what that all angels were there to help me help her. We didn't have the pain meds we do now that had concentrated morphine in drops to put under the tongue or patches to deliver the medication over two or three days.

So the angels came through, and I got her IV inserted. I gave her the prescribed dose of morphine very slowly. "Oh, Lord," I whispered with all sincerity, "please don't let this poor little lady die this minute. Just give her rest from her pain and then when she is resting comfortable take her in Your time, so these kids don't think they killed her by asking for more pain medication for her."

Then I taped down the IV needle and sat with her as she began to breathe easier. The tenseness in her tiny frame began to subside. The girls' eyeballs were peering around the corner. As they saw her begin to ease up, they were brave enough to come back in her room. They gathered around her and gently pat on her and cooed, "That's right, Mom. Now you can go to sleep and rest. We love you, Mom."

I gathered supplies and went to the living room. I decided against troubling her for a blood pressure check. It didn't matter. Her respirations were steady and even, but everyone knew it wouldn't be long. They told me they were comfortable being alone with her. They were afraid of her dying. They just didn't want her to suffer anymore. So I headed back to the office.

They lived out in the country; it gave me a dose of commanding views and time to think and thank God for always being with us and

88

with these families and all these patients. It was nearly summer and warm sunlight hit my left arm as I held it out the window to feel the rays. I wished and prayed for her to know warmth from above, peace in the process, the amazing White Light that many speak of, and for those children to always remember they helped her stay home in that dear little bedroom that made her so happy.

CHAPTER 12

PRAYING THE NICEST LITTLE PRAYERS

Bill and Betty lived way out between two little towns northeast of where our office was located. So I wanted to try to not forget any of the supplies I needed to take with me for my visit with him that day.

We had only just admitted Bill to our hospice care that week and he was rapidly declining. He didn't weigh much and still he had a strong will. He didn't want to be put in a hospital bed unless it was absolutely necessary.

"You girls may think me foolish, but I want to stay in the same bed me and my wife have shared for years. Betty lies down by me gently and I sleep better with her at my side. She also gently strokes my hand and says stuff I like to hear. She's always praying the nicest little prayers for me. She's always done that. She'll pray, 'Lord, help Bill sleep a deep peaceful sleep this night. Lord, bless Bill's bones with rest and no pain this night. Blessed Jesus, give Bill a dream full of peace and joy. Sweet Lord, touch my Bill's spirit with Your Spirit so he can be reminded that You hold him and love him so much.' You know? Like that all the time, real sweet and soft, and I fall asleep with those prayers and the cross with Jesus on it tucked 'neath my pillow."

How on earth are you going to try to talk someone out of their bed with that most earnest request?! We decided to wait until it was "absolutely necessary."

She was a tough ole' girl. She didn't show any fear. She was focused on giving him the calmest, smoothest, most pain-free transition that could be known. She was so careful to administer his pain meds where she was meeting the need but not giving him too much. She gently turned him over to check to make sure his posture was helping his aching bones to know the most profitable position. She kept the smallest fan on in the hallway to give him a little breeze but didn't let it hit him in the face. She fixed fresh homemade soups full of nutrients but thin enough for him to swallow "only what he wants" amounts. She let in the visitors that he wanted to see and no one else. And she cautioned them to not stay over five minutes at a time.

One night I got the call just before midnight. "Could you come be with us? I think I know all the right things to do, but he thinks we should have one of you girls with us, and they said you were on call tonight. I'm so sorry to bother you."

"It's no bother. I'll be dressed in a flash and head your way," I answered back.

During my drive up there, the dark sky was glittery and showing off stars I thought were just made up. Millions of shining lights seemingly singing and liking very much that they were the stars they were created to be. Silly, happy stars.

I pulled into the driveway and made my way to the back utility room door so as not to make much noise with the front room door.

She was sitting with him on the side of the bed. His breathing was indeed very low and shallow, but still he was aware and acknowledged my arrival. He moved a finger wave and tried to wink.

"I'm going to get a teaspoon of ice chips," his wife announced in a soft tone.

Then she tugged on my jacket to look at her. She was motioning me to follow.

"He's close but he's hurting. Can we give him just a little of that pain medicine the doctor sent out? I just don't want to push him over the edge," she asked.

"That's what the doctor wanted, him to be comfortable; you are not pushing him over the edge doing that. It's a very small dose, and I don't want you to worry about that at all. Would you like for me to give this dose to him for you?" I asked still in whispering tones.

"No, I want to give it to him. I've done all this up till now, and I'm not quitting now."

We tiptoed back into the bedroom. He was taking his last breath. She gathered him up into her arms and softly said all those prayers again that he had told me about. I stood by her and told her as she finished I would be in the kitchen if she would like some time alone with him.

"Oh, no, that's okay. He's gone now. He must've known I was concerned about that last dose and took care of things for me. Just like him. Bless him. Oh my, I'm so thankful for no more bone pain for him, but I'm not sure I'll survive my broken heart."

I held her while she cried. Then she dried her tears with her Kleenex she pulled out of her jeans pocket and said, "Let's make some coffee while we wait for the funeral home to arrive. You go call them, and I'll get the information that they'll want ready."

Somewhere deep inside I see some people pull up an energy and a strength that's rolling around with grief, shock, and sorrow at those moments and just do what needs to be done.

I drove home looking back at those sassy singing stars. I pray when my time comes I know someone like her to sit by me and say those same kinds of prayers.

CHAPTER 13

DON'T UPSET THIS FAMILY!

The Howards were a really proud bunch of people. They didn't really want strangers in the house helping them with their dad, Mr. Howard, but they admitted they needed the help.

I was a little nervous—not so much about them as I was about him. I had heard tales that he would bite your head off and hand it to you on a platter. Yikes!

His heart wasn't obliging by staying strong enough to pump the blood around his body anymore like it was suppose to do. He wasn't a candidate for a transplant, even though he had told more than one big city doctor he could afford it if he did want one.

His heart specialist warned me. "Don't upset this family, and don't piss him off either!"

Well!! That's one way of asking a nurse to visit a patient!

I mustered up my courage and headed in their direction. It was one of those houses that you had to call ahead of time so someone could open a big gate. Sometimes it's a big gate and more often a concrete driveway or a dirt road, but the same needs are waiting inside.

I was trying to be very professional and not look like Ellie Mae Clampett gone to the city the first time I walked in there. The artwork on the walls must have cost more than my house, I thought. Never in my life had I walked on such plush carpet. The man who let me in asked if he could take my bag.

"No, sir, I need it when I visit Mr. Howard, but thanks all the same." All the same? Oh, shoot! That sounded almost hillbilly, I thought.

Well, I had never seen a bedroom that big either. The hospital bed looked like a dollhouse toy. But, as much as he could, he tried to look very important and all-knowing. I could see how frail he was, and I decided to be forgiving if he was mean.

He wasn't at all! In fact, he introduced himself and smiled. He asked me all kinds of questions about hospice. He wanted to know how I decided to be a hospice nurse, what college I had attended, what town I lived in, and all kinds of information.

I tried to answer every question and be very polite and not show any fear. The longer I stayed with him the easier I felt. He made me feel welcome. He offered me a soft drink or tea as if I were his neighbor. Smart man.

After I finished my assessment and instructions and time for him to ask questions, he requested I have a seat next to his bed. His son and daughter scurried to get the nearest chair, and then they exited the room and closed the doors.

"I suppose you've heard about my reputation. I've been known to be a mean SOB in my day. I'm not sure why I ever thought that was the way to handle myself or my family or my business. I always wanted to be in charge and for everyone to believe I knew exactly what I was doing and not to cross me. I don't have a better answer unless it's that I may have been insecure and thought if I growled it'd go better. As you can tell, I've been thinking lately about all this and have had discussions with my children and some of my partners and apologized to all of them. They have been gracious.

"I've seen my grandmother lately in my dreams and I believe no

94

one in life has ever loved me as much as that woman did. There is where I found my decency again, in the spot down deep that she created for me and I had left behind.

"So, now what I want for you and me is to have a relationship where I tell you what's going on with me and you answer the questions that can be answered and you always be honest when you don't know the answer. Is that a workable deal for you young lady?"

"Yes, sir, it is," I honestly replied.

Sometime later I got back to the hospital and halfway down the hallway. One of the other nurses caught me and said, "Hey! How did that go? Was he living up to his reputation, you poor little lamb?" she asked as she laughed.

I stopped, turned, and replied, "He was a gentleman." And then I went to my cubby hole and made a new chart for him.

Isn't it funny how we think we always know how a very first meeting with someone might turn out and, low and behold, it is totally different than we imagined? Oh, that I may always be surprised!!

Nice people sometimes need to say a mean thing or two and mean people can turn soft.

CHAPTER 14

COON HOUNDS AND CHICKENS

When I got the address to this place I thought I had better throw bread crumbs along the gravel road going in. Then I noticed on my way to the house that there were stray dogs that would have eaten them. My ancient car phone back then just lit up a message like, "Yeah, right! No service." And then it died.

I drove up on this pitiful mobile home that looked like it had seen better days in the '50s. Coon dogs and hound dogs were lying in dug-up ditches under the weeping willow tree. Chickens were scratching for any hope of a bug not too far from the front gate.

"Oh, Lord, give me courage," I prayed as I walked gingerly up to the lean-to porch. Those dogs didn't get up. They just raised their heads, looked at me, and then fell back over.

"Hello? Hello? Anybody here?" I weakly hollered out while knocking.

"Sure, Honey. Come on in here outta that nasty ole' heat. We can't hear none too good with that water cooler whining in the living room window. Ma hates the dad-blasted thing, so she stays in the back bedroom. She likes it warmer since she's up and lost all that weight the past two months.

"Maw! Maw! That nurse lady I told you about is here. She come to check on you like the doctor asked her to and she needs to see about ya," she announced.

"Maw" tried to open her eyes and peek out at me and decided it wasn't worth the effort and shut them again.

"Come in, Honey. I'm too tired to get up. This bed's done taken to my shape, and it's hard to crawl out of unless there's a fire or some other threat to force me."

I inched my way through the crowded room and found a spot on a vegetable crate from the feed store and put my lab coat over it. I made myself a suitable spot to look her over.

I explained why I was there and that we hope to help keep her comfortable during this time. I assured her that I would try to meet any need she had.

With that she opened one eyeball and sheepishly smiled and said, "What I need is a man about thirty years old and for him to have a fat bank account and we'd high tail it outta here and go to some swanky hotel in Tulsie-Town and turn on the air conditioner and have us a cocktail and live it up till this ticker quit. But with my luck, I wouldn't make it out of the driveway."

Just then I thought to myself, "Never, ever in my life of nursing, have I ever been bored! Period."

That made my day. I inched up closer to her, took her hand, and said, "What kind of cocktail?"

She giggled so hard she peed the bed; I had to give her a sponge bath.

I finished my work there and headed out the door and through the gate. I told the dogs good-bye and waved the chickens away from the car. In front of me stood a goat looking like he wanted to make this visit even more memorable with a head butt. I got in my car and didn't look back till my phone alerted me that she was in the land of the living again.

97

I could have gotten to know that great little lady even better, but she passed away before I could make my next visit. The other nurses said she didn't say much to them. Of course, they looked more professional than I did. Maybe she didn't think they would think her way of 'thinking' would be as much fun as I did. They would have.

CHAPTER 15

GIANT GEESE AND TINY COPPERHEADS

Speaking of driving in the boonies, you have to understand that to some people in some counties, what I think of the boonies is their local neighborhood, their local hangout. But, when I started following the directions to this new place, I was concerned about finding my way out again.

The house I pulled up to was in sad shape. She was sort of leaning to the east and hadn't been painted in maybe thirty or forty years. I gathered up my stethoscope and bag and opened the car door when five giant geese ran around from the back of the house to greet me.

I eased my way through them, protecting myself with my bag to get to the front door, speaking as big and mean as possible, "Down goose! Back goose! Shoo!"

Once inside I found my patient right inside the front door in her loaned hospital bed. Her hair was as white as snow and she had cloudy blue eyes that had cataracts. She was quick to tell me she couldn't see me well enough to make out what I looked like but that it didn't matter and to come on in.

"Please don't hurt my geese. I heard them fussing with you. They are good watch dog geese. And they eat the baby copperheads in the yard," she proudly announced.

"Copperheads?" I squeaked out.

She needed a bandage changed, her blood drawn for a lab test, and a bed bath since the aide was ill. There was a huge, ancient pot-belly stove just a couple of feet from the foot of her bed, and there were the nicest pictures of Jesus on the walls from calendars of years gone by.

"You can go fetch the water from the kitchen sink. There's a pan in that hallway by the bathroom door. And when you finish with it you can take it out back and put that water on the flowers. We don't waste a drop of water." She spoke as loudly as she possibly could.

"And while you're in the kitchen, you can get a piece of that 'fat-back' out of the 'frigerator and use it on my sore on my elbow. It'll draw out the infection the doctor thinks is there. Now, I know he thinks he knows best with the medication he sent, but too much of that stuff will kill ya. I like the old ways better."

"Yes, ma'am. I understand. My grandma felt the same way. We had to force her to go to the doctor, and she didn't trust a one of them. She said—oh well, anyway she wouldn't take antibiotics either. But since the doctor wanted me to clean your wound with some peroxide and iodine, I better stick to his order."

The best thing about spending time with someone to give them something as personal as a bath is that you get to see their skin and how it looks, and if there are sore places in hiding, tiny broken open areas, rashes, redness, bruises, and the like. So, we were talking and I was gently examining and gently washing her very fragile skin and then when I turned her over I discovered a six-inch tiny black petrified snake in the bed with her. I neither jumped, screamed, nor said a word. It was dead and wasn't hurting anything. Poor little fellow didn't know he would get squashed up there.

I took him out of the bed and gently laid him on the chair next to me. When I finished her bath time I took him outside and put him on a rock. Who knows? Maybe geese eat snake jerky?

100

We had many visits over the months to follow, and her elbow healed up nicely. But her oldest son came from out of state one day and decided she needed to be in a nursing home closer to him where he could see her more often. She took her photos of Jesus and put them in her room. That was what she said she had planned to do anyway. I hope so. She said she was happy that she could see her son more often. But she cried when she thought of leaving her geese.

I went home and petted every pet I owned and thanked God for my eyesight and my floor. I checked under my bed for little snakes.

CHAPTER 16

MEETING 'RATTY'

I was asked to go see Fred, an elderly gentleman who had had abdominal surgery and needed to have his dressing changed and educated on how to prevent infection and how to re-dress the bandages, among other things.

Fred and his family didn't live too far from town in a semi-rural setting. There were cars that had been decaying for quite some time in the front and side yards, and I suspected even in the backyard. A variety of animals were all over the property, and they all stopped what they were doing when I got out of the car. I was trying to sum up my chances of making a run for it when one of the sons stepped out on the concrete steps and said, "Come on in! Daddy's expected you. I'll guard ya while you get inside!"

Good.

When I got inside, I knew I should have brought my soap. Lord have mercy! These precious people were living among collections of collected garage sale finds and they weren't sure where to put them or when they would need them. They were keeping them handy in the living room and the kitchen and the bedroom...and the bathroom! All the dishes—I was guessing here—they owned were dirty, and I could not find dish soap or hand soap or even laundry soap to wash my hands before starting. So I searched for some hand cleaner from my bag; I was afraid to put it down! But there in a little bedroom Fred was lying in his bed with all his grown kids circling the bed. His wife was standing next to him with a football helmet on. "We are proud to see you, nurse," she said, greeting me.

"Don't mind my helmet. I been having seizures and falling over and so I decided it might save my noggin if I keep this helmet on," she said while patting it.

"Oh, that's a good idea," I replied.

Her dear little fella in the bed was so very thin and as weak as a kitten. He grinned at me and said, "I hope you can get that tape off my belly without pulling my entire hide off like they dern ner done in the hospital."

"I'll try to be very gentle. I've got some great stuff in this bag that will help with that," I proudly shared like I had gold nuggets in there.

Everyone wanted to watch the changing of this bandage so they remained in position around the bed. I began opening up my sterile gloves and gauze pads and all the other items I needed. I had made a temporary sterile field at the bottom of his mattress since there wasn't a clean table in sight.

Just about the time I was ready to start peeling off the old bandage, a rat the size of a small Chihuahua came out from underneath the bed. I jumped up on that bed and knocked everything across the room.

All of them started laughing. The wife said, "Oh, don't be afraid of 'Ratty.' He don't bother anything much, and he lays under the bed pretty quiet most of the time."

It did take me a minute or two to get my bearings, but I was constantly watching out for Ratty's return with one eye.

"Well, thank you much, nurse. Come on back anytime you want. We will watch out after Mommy and Daddy, and we'll call you down there at that hospital if we need anything before you come back," The oldest said while I was running to the car.

They helped him get that surgical wound healed without infection, and I bought them some more soap and sneaked it into the bathroom and kitchen. I got used to Ratty—well, almost.

CHAPTER 17

TAKING CARE OF BUSINESS

John wasn't too happy about having to stop work long enough to go to the hospital for all the tests the doctor ordered. And he certainly wasn't pleased about the bronchoscope needed to get down his "guzzle" to get a pinch of a biopsy to see what that was in his lung showing up on the x-ray.

But his daughter was insisting he find out what they were dealing with so they could make decisions. He thought the sun rose and set with this daughter so he agreed. She had practically raised herself, he told me during that first visit. Her mother had passed on early in her life. So it was just the two of them.

They lived far away from the big city hospital. I went down one highway, down a county line road, and then through a cattle guard gate to find their place. I backed up, but not too close, to a creek and a bunch of shady trees, with cows lying down under them. They were chewing their cuds like they were making some kind of commercial for happy cows.

I grew up in the country so I always liked going to a place out of town to make a visit. It was spring and the dogwoods and redbuds were bursting with blooms and scattering color all along that creek bed. Birds were chattering up a storm when I got out of the car, and squirrels were chasing each other around the older, larger oak trees. I could see deer at the back of the pasture on full alert. The air was clean after another spring storm the night before.

"Well, are you going to come in the house or stay out here all day long with these critters?" he asked while holding open his living room screen door.

"Oh, I'm sorry I was taking so long. I was admiring your beautiful place here. Does that creek ever flood and cause you trouble? Because if it doesn't, you got paradise going on here." I said while making my way up to the entrance.

"Well, when I was younger, we had some doozy storms and flooded us a couple of times, but nothing we couldn't handle. Since then we raised the house we brought out here up on those foundation stones and we stay dry. The animals move up to higher ground and they stay dry and safe.

"But that's neither here nor there. Come on in and let's get acquainted. My daughter said the doctor was sending you out here to take blood from this new port they put up here by my collar bone. You must know from talking to him I got me this lung cancer and I've never smoked a cigarette in my life. Go figure! Well, there's going to be a lot of those treatments, and my veins aren't too great, so they decided to put in this contraption to make it easier on me to give me chemo and take my blood or if they need to give me blood. You probably already know all this don't ya, young lady?"

"Well, yes sir, most of it. But I wanted to know how you feel about all this. It must have been quite a shock having lung cancer when you never smoked."

"That's right. But my daughter says it happens. Some people just get it. And you can't sit around and belly ache about it all day and all night. That's a waste of good energy and time. Person needs to get about their business of doing whatever the plan involves to get you better or to at least try.

"That daughter of mine needs to believe that there's hope I can make 'er. She's been disappointed before with losing her mother. I gotta fight this tooth and toenail so she knows I tried."

I had all the necessary equipment to access the port, draw the blood, and flush the line after. I finished our visit and put the tubes in my safe blood sample carrying kit and got ready to go.

"Say, young lady, I was wondering if you ever saw anyone with my kind of lung cancer survive?" he asked while holding his sweat-stained hat and scratching his head.

"I've read about it. So, yes, there are survivors from this kind of lung cancer. It's a fight, but some do make it on the other side of the fight," I assured him with a hint of caution.

"Thank you. I'll give that positive note to the girl. I know she's nearing forty now, but she's still my girl. Thank you for coming out here. God bless ya for what you do."

Then he waved his cap at me and walked around the house toward the creek.

In all honesty, there weren't many successes I had read about, but he needed some hope. And some days a little hope can go a long ways. God bless us all with an abundance of hope!

CHAPTER 18

DON'T BE FLAPPING YOUR JAW!

They were the last two surviving sisters in the family. Beth was dying from cancer and Mary, the older sister, was caring for her. They lived in Beth's home and so Mary brought her husband who was also ailing along with her. They were staying "as long as it took."

"Okay, lookie here. You need to remember we aren't exactly spring chickens that you're dealing with and trying to teach stuff to, okay? You got that? I can't remember where I parked my car at Walmart so easy does it, kiddo, on too much info. I mean, I'm willing to do whatever needs to be done for Beth but just remember what I'm telling ya is all I'm saying."

"Oh, Becki, don't pay any attention to all that fussing about too much information. She's the smartest of all us kids and pretends not to be. And she acts all tough and has a heart as big as Dallas. She would give ya the shirt off her back if you needed it and look how they up and moved to town to be with me while Henry's none too well neither.

"Anyhow, we'll make it just fine. Look at this quilt she brought

108

me to dress up my bed and make it all fancy for you nurses to see! She's a seamstress. She is and famous for her pickled beets. And no one would ever know she went to college and got a business degree when women didn't do that all that much when she went and did it."

"Oh, good grief. You're telling her too much, Beth. This nurse just came to see how much swellin' is in your legs. Don't be flapping your jaw so much." And with that she pulled back the covers. Her swelling was pretty serious. Her skin was weeping from all the water she was holding. And her toes were turning purple. The tumors in her abdomen and pelvis region had grown faster than her doctor had originally anticipated. I acted like it wasn't so bad and pulled the covers back up.

"Would you like for me to wrap your legs in some soft gauze and put fresh padding underneath?" I asked.

"Oh, don't you bother. Mary will do it. She likes being all important and being in charge of my care. We're making it okay. We are just taking this one day at a time. And today my little preacher from our home town where we grew up about thirty miles north of here came out and visited and prayed for us. He's a nice young man and has made a difference in our weekly visits. He's so positive and kind and we don't think he fully understands how serious this is and the time left, but we like him and his little stories he tells and we think its better not to trouble him with too much truth. One of our members called and told us that when he found out Sister Ruth was failing; he got all serious and depressed and didn't have much to say when he visited her. So we're trying to spare him."

At times it seems like I've traveled back in time, to the '40s or '50s, perhaps, with some of these patients and their lives. Not everyone has a television in every room and on all the time. Some people turn on the radio or just visit with family and friends. You might see old dishes and older furniture and aprons and someone soaking beans and making cornbread and doilies on the arms of the chairs. The dead giveaway are the cell phones some child will buy for a parent. When it would ring it would scare all three of them, and they take a few minutes to decide who would answer it and how. Mary is the most educated, so she takes on the duty.

She makes another decision and turns the phone to silent.

All three of them smile.

"Oftentimes we think it's so important to know all the latest information out there about computers and phones and televisions and the like. And don't get me started on trying to play an old movie I bought.

"But some of us are happy and contented in knowing we don't have to know every last bit of it. Our kids or our grandkids will help us if we really need it."

At this point they didn't need it. They were happy in making her last days as much like the old place as possible. Homemade biscuits with jam were offered to Beth by Mary with scrambled eggs if she wanted it.

Chicken and dumplings were on the menu. Sliced beefsteak tomatoes were mentioned with mouth-watering homemade macaroni and cheese baked to bubbly perfection from the oven. Yeast rolls were made on Sunday with the fried chicken they alternated with meat loaf and sometimes a small roast with potatoes and carrots, all lovingly prepared by Mary.

Mary sat me down one day at the tiny kitchen table while doing dishes and said, "You need to eat just one bite or two of macaroni and cheese. I know you're watching your cholesterol, but you ought step out of that box every now and then and have a biscuit or a slice of chocolate cake fresh out of the oven with a dip of vanilla ice cream."

So I did. Henry sat with me and we talked about when he was a boy and what he ate for dinner.

Mary went in the room with Beth and they were whispering and laughing a little.

Who would have known death was at the door?

CHAPTER 19

MINK COAT AND TENNIS SHOES

Another patient in the outpatient oncology unit caught my eye the day she waltzed in and loudly announced, "Hey, good morning everyone. Where's Betty? I need her to check out this chest tube!"

She was wearing a hip-length mink coat, tennis shoes, and a multi-colored silk scarf tied on her head. She also had giant diamonds on both hands.

"Oh, boy!" I thought. "We have a character here!"

I told her Betty was in a room with the doctor seeing a patient and she would be right out. She nodded and looked me over, sizing me up.

"I'm working part-time here while she finishes her master's. Can I do anything for you?"

"No thanks, kiddo, I'm attached to Betty. But thanks for asking." She smiled.

Later Betty told me she was only about thirty years old and had been all over the world traveling and refused to believe that cancer was going to stop her. She listened to advice the doctors had given her about staying in the United States while on treatments. But now the cancer was back with a vengeance, and one lung wasn't doing too well; the other one had the chest tube in to drain a bloody mixture of fluids.

As the weeks and months went by, she began to come in quieter and with less energy. Then one day she had to be admitted to the in-patient ward. She was dying. She had accepted me along the way and Betty told her I "knew God," so she had the nurse upstairs call down and ask for me to come up and pray with her.

Up those back stairs I climbed and started praying ahead of time. When I reached her room she was lying very still and looking out the east window where some sunshine was washing her window with light. She had two sisters with her. One was blowing her nose and trying not to cry out loud. The other one was sitting with her head in her hands.

I went closer and she reached for my hand. "I don't know how to pray. My sisters have been praying, and a nice minister came in and prayed with us. I was thinking the more prayers the better." All of this was coming out of her with great effort but just above a whisper.

I pulled a pillow off the wide window sill and threw it down on the floor next to the head of her bed. She gave me her hand and her sisters came and stood on either side of me, now openly weeping. I asked God to give her peace, the peace that passes all understanding. I asked God to help her know her angels were near and watching for her, with her. I asked God to help her transition be smooth and for her to have visions in her sleep of where she was going. And I asked God to help those sisters to have all they needed in this time as well.

I kissed her pale thin hand and excused myself after hugging her sisters. I walked to the end of the hallway and one of them called me back with urgency.

As I entered her room, I knew what had happened. She was gone. But the expression on her face was so serene. No more scowl, no more furrowed brow—just peace.

CHAPTER 20

WE'LL BE OKAY

I was heading out of town to visit a family who were caring for their mom. She was dying with kidney failure. The directions were along the line of, "You know where the highway divides a few miles east of town? Well, bear toward the right and you'll be headed south. When you reach the first stop sign in our community you need to go left and then turn right at the big red barn that sits two miles west of that last turn."

"Okie dokie!" I thought.

But they were really good directions.

When I got to the street address and house number painted on the curb, I glanced toward the house and thought, "Oh, boy, here we go. Give me your patience and kindness, Lord."

The grass was up to my knees. The paint on the house was peeling, and the roof looked like there might be leaking somewhere upstairs.

I glanced up at the sight of movement and I began to see kids appearing all over the place. One boy with copper red hair of about six or seven came running from the nearby Laundromat screaming,

"Hey, nurse lady! Over here! I'll show ya the front door and how to get in!"

The thing was I had been circling the house trying to figure out which door to knock on. Nothing really looked like a front door.

Then here came another child of about four or five years old, cotton-topped head, skipping and jumping in the grass that nearly swallowed him up. "Hey, nurse lady, let me show you. Let me!" A girl with long red braids and maybe close to ten was heading my way as well and announced with authority, "I'll show her. You goofballs stay back!"

So all of them reached me about the same time and all wanted to take my hands or my arms and lead me to the faded blue door where we made our entrance.

"You kids scatter on out of here. Let that poor woman get in here to see Me-Maw." And they did.

Me-Maw was in a twin bed in the corner of the darkened room with a wedding circle quilt lightly lying across her feet and legs. She had clean braided grayish red hair and a crisp white pillowcase embroidered with Dutch maids dancing with milk buckets. Her flannel sheets were clean as well and the room was full of her grown children, all with red or blonde hair, all standing at attention.

"We understand, ma'am, that you are here to help us with our mom and we want you to know we appreciate that kindness. But, with no disrespect, we want to keep her here with us. She don't like them hospitals too much. She wants to be here with us and we can make sure she's comfortable. She likes it when she can see these kids, and we let her little poodle doggie up on the bed every now and then and he licks her hand and makes her smile. We couldn't bring him up to that hospital. We can learn anything you want to teach us 'bout her care." He politely and tenderly spoke with such admiration and love for her. I think he was fearful that I was going to suggest they move her back to the hospital.

They all were nodding in agreement.

"I can cook for all of us," one daughter announced.

114

"And I can watch after all the grandkids," another offered.

"And I used to be an aide in a nursing home, and I know how to turn her and keep her clean and wash her dentures if she ever wants them back in there. She won't take her medication anymore and the doctor said not to bother with it. He told us and her she could stay here if she let you come see about all of us," the youngest of the three said.

Even with a brief assessment it was evident their mother did not have many hours left—possibly days, but I doubted it. Her feet were already blue and her knee caps were mottled. Her skin temperature was very cool to touch but her back was warm with fever. She was semi-comatose and not showing any evidence of discomfort. She had quit eating or drinking about three days before. She was in or nearing kidney failure the doctor suspected.

I sat down in the kitchen with them and told them what a great job they were doing. I told them what they already knew. She didn't have long, but couldn't give them an exact hour like so many ask for. I told them to continue exactly what they were doing, being with her. I told them that their quiet hushed tones were a good idea and that gently stroking her arm or reassuring her of their presence was also nice. I explained about the active dying process and gave them some handouts. I asked them if they would like for me to stay a while longer.

The youngest replied, "We've been with our daddy, too, when he passed on, and I've been with a few at the nursing home. I think we will be fine, but we appreciate you being kind enough to ask us. We'll be okay."

"I totally agree. No one could do a better job than all of you together like this. I know she is so proud of you," I said.

I left them our number and headed out the faded blue door. All the kids came back running my way. "Hey, nurse lady, come back again and see us!" they hollered in unison and waved above the grass.

How many times does the good Lord remind me, you can't judge a home by the way the house looks.

CHAPTER 21

THE GREATER GIFT

This was another one of those directions where I was hoping I had written it all down right. "Go to the third stop sign after the first stop light heading west on Elm, then turn left on Fourth and go to that house just on the corner that is green. You can't miss it."

Well, they were right. Her sister was giving me the directions while she was screaming in the background any corrections she thought might help. There wasn't a driveway so I just pulled up in front by the curb. There wasn't a garage either but just a little green square house of about 800 square feet or so. Man oh man! I could barely get in the door due to all the stuff they had piled up next to the entrance. There were old magazines, dirty clothes, books, ancient encyclopedias—you name it.

I introduced myself and she glowingly replied, "Well, welcome and sit down here next to my bed, and let's get acquainted before you start in on this stump.

"Helen, get 'er some of that coffee, and see if there's a donut left in that bag that Dorothy Mae brought in earlier."

"Oh, no thank you. I had two cups of coffee already, and I'm trying to keep off the donuts lately, but I thank you kindly for the offer."

Her sister was grinning and winked at me as she moved around from her sister's bed and started folding a load of towels and putting them on an ironing board set up next to the dining table that looked like it was being used for storing more stuff.

"Well, let me give you some history if they haven't already filled you in. I had my first leg cut off about a year ago due to my blood veins aren't worth two cents. Then my second leg started actin' up and my foot was turning black, and they had to up and cut it off too. So there you have it. They tell me I might be okay for a few years but that my heart ain't none too perfect neither. So, we'll get this new stump healed up and we'll watch our soap operas and eat some donuts and read some of those *Reader's Digest* books I've been savin'.

"Oh, and I forgot to mention, even though my leg's gone, she still thinks she's here. I feel pain in that foot that they cut off with my leg. Isn't that funny? The first time that happened with my other amputation I thought I was going crazy. They ought a tell a person about that before surgery and not wait till later. That's dern spooky."

I got out my supplies to change her dressing and balanced them on the ironing board and made a sterile field and went to work teaching both of them how to do this themselves. They didn't miss a thing.

"Yep. That's right. I 'member that from the last one. Yep. That's right, nurse. See that, sister? You can't wipe your nose or anything while we're doing this once you put on those gloves."

Again, her sister looked up at me and winked.

I left them my new bar of soap I had in the car since they couldn't find theirs. But I left with a greater gift.

Driving home I thought about my high school days in home economics class. I had the nicest teacher. She was so kind and patient with me. I couldn't ever get it right when I was suppose to thread that sewing machine to make a dress and, when I did finish it, the whole class was trying not to laugh. Then I burned the hotcakes we were making...or was it muffins? One day she gently whispered, "Maybe you'll be good in typing."

I'm just glad I took that only job in the paper that spring of 1971 as a nurse's aide in the nursing home. It fit like a glove.

CHAPTER 22

THE FEEL OF A HOUSE

The neighboring town to the west of us didn't have a home health or hospice office up and running yet when I went to work at the one in our town. So we started seeing their patients as well. I liked driving over there and getting my brain all lined out ahead of time on my schedule and driving plan.

His house sits up on top of a hill facing the south. There were pine and fruit trees, lilac and Rose of Sharon bushes, but I didn't see any flowers. Bernie greeted me at the door and welcomed me inside. There was a sad and strange feel about the house. Everything seemed clean and in order but there was just something about the *feel* of it.

He was such a quiet, kind man. He was grateful and thankful he didn't have to drive back to the big city hospital to have this drainage tube from his side that drained his one good kidney cleaned and flushed with sterile fluids and redressed.

His dog, Shep, watched me from a safe distance at the entry to his bedroom.

"He's kind of shy, but he's a real good dog. We both been a little

119

on the sad side since my wife passed away a few months ago. Mae was the light of this house. She was always humming some little church tune, and the oven always had something baking in it that made the whole house smell like a bakery. She had flower beds all around the house and kept fresh flowers in her antique crystal vase over there in that window that connects the kitchen to the dining room. Her favorite was her iris. She hated it that they didn't bloom all spring and summer. She had all colors of them and talked to them like they heard her. I dug them up and gave them to her best friend when she died. She's going to plant them in her flower bed close to her house so she can feel like she still has her close by. I didn't want to see them bloom again.

"We didn't have any kids due to her female trouble, but she never let on like she thought she was any less of a woman not being a mother. She mothered everyone and everything. We were married forty-eight years. We were planning a big celebration for our fiftieth. I'm sorry we didn't make that one. I got her picture of when she was in high school right over there on that end table by the couch. I like to look at it and sometimes I talk to her. Shep lays there on that rug next to me and looks at me like I've lost all my brains and turns around and looks for her.

"I miss a lot of things with her passing. She spoiled me, and I knew she did, but I don't think I ever told her how much I appreciated all she did. She acted like she was excited every time I walked into the house, like she hadn't seen me in days. She was funny that way. And she ironed all my shirts, and they didn't really need it after we got that new washer and dryer, but she did anyway.

"She made me a special dessert every night but made me walk every morning before work to help keep me healthy, she said. She would sneak out some mornings after getting the clothes out of the washer and hang them on our old clothesline. I scolded her and told her she needed to use that expensive dryer, but she said the sheets smelled sweeter after getting all that fresh country air blown through them. I thought that was nonsense.

120

"It was too hard for me to see all her stuff here, so I had her girlfriend come and get her clothes and shoes and purses and perfume... and...."

He stopped talking and looked out the big picture window facing the fruit trees.

"I'll be all right. I thank you for letting me talk about some of that. My family and hers can't stand it, and so we don't discuss her when we're together. But I like to hear her name. I like it when her best friend comes and we share stories about her. Sure, we cry some, but we laugh some too. She's a nice woman. She tries to make me feel better by baking a cake every now and then. I take it and say thanks but I only eat a small piece and give Shep a bite. She doesn't cook as well as Mae did.

"But me and Shep won't say nothing, will we, boy?"

I finished up my duties and asked if he would like for me to do anything else.

"No, but I thank you for that offer. I'm here all day, and I try to tidy up like she did and keep it all nice and clean. I talk to Shep an awful lot. I know it sounds crazy but I think he understands me. He follows me around while I'm doing laundry or washing up my few dishes. Don't write that down in your paperwork about Shep or they'll send a padded wagon after me." And then he smiled for the first time.

We continued our visits with him until the doctor took out the tube and discharged him from our service. Those last few visits the house "personality" became a little lighter and brighter each time. And, on one of those visits, I noticed a vase full of multicolored irises on the coffee table. Shep was wagging his tail, and my patient's color was better.

Six months later I saw him downtown where he lived. He was all dressed up in a starched white shirt, wearing a new hat, and holding hands with a lady. He stopped me and said, "I want you to meet someone."

I think Mae sent her his way. Don't you?

CHAPTER 23

BARNS AND SILOS, PIGS AND COWS

I had just begun writing an article for the local newspaper about what patients teach me when I got the assignment to go see this fellow named Bud way out in the country who had a heart attack recently. His doctor had him on bed rest for a few days until his strength returned.

The drive out there was blessing me with scenery of silos, fifty-year-old barns, dairy cows, and hog pens with piglets running around. It was April and a fresh spontaneous downpour had just stopped filling creek beds and making frogs dance a jig. Every Spring I would see these show-off lilacs and forsythia bushes seeming so proud to show their stuff. Daffodils lined the walk to the door, and I could hear a newborn calf bawling behind me in a little fenced in spot for him and his mother was licking him and watching out to see if I was friend or foe.

Bud's charming, "well loved by all" wife let me inside and headed to get me some lemonade while I sat with him to do his paperwork and check him over. He had his large leather-bound Bible on the coffee table in front of the couch where he was propped up on feather pillows.

I worked with his daughter-in-law and knew him so we talked about his kids, grandkids, his farm, and then finally his heart. He didn't let on like he was concerned at all. "We trust in the Lord for each day. We're thankful for all the goodness we know and have always known," he said while nodding thanks to his wife for the cool drinks.

We went over the medications, signs, symptoms of any trouble showing up, safety measures, phone numbers, and vital signs: the whole kit and caboodle.

He was so humble and gracious and was well known in the community as such a godly man. He was always doing for others.

He asked me to pray for him before I left. Then he opened his Bible and flipped through thin, worn pages till he found the spot he was looking for and said, "Here, Becki, this is the verse I think God wants you to know."

I thanked him and hugged him and his wife.

I put the verse in my nurse bag and tried to focus on driving.

A few months later he had another heart episode and had to have surgery. When I saw his daughter-in-law at work she stopped me in the hallway.

"Oh, Becki, I have to tell you something!"

"What?!" I thought he had died in surgery or something.

"I went to see Bud in ICU last night. He pulled me close to him and said, 'Tell Becki to keep writing her articles.'"

I had chills racing up and down my whole body. I was so very humbled and honored that he would even think of me. I know she couldn't help but see my condition.

"No, he said you are supposed to keep writing your articles. That's what he said. I don't know about you, but I wasn't expecting those to be his words right after surgery!"

I just stood there like a zombie and shook my head. Then I thanked her and turned and went to my car. Down deep in the scary recesses of my bag where I kept all I thought I needed on a moment's notice at a patient's home, I found the wrinkled piece of paper with the scripture verse. I held it to my chest.

Much later when his time did arrive to "head home," I chose to sit in the back of the quaint country church he loved. It was packed. So many people and family and neighbors and church members wanted to be there. One of his sons got up and told all of us that his dad didn't want any bragging on him. He just wanted people to praise God.

Just like him.

CHAPTER 24

BEYOND STATISTICS

When I was in nursing school the instructors were always telling about facts and figures with diseases and the like. There were all kinds of statistics.

I wasn't interested as much in the numbers as I was in the person in the bed, the person in the chemo chair, the person standing next to the bed, and all that went with that. I liked getting to know the cat and seeing wedding photos, and hearing about their military service or about the time the tornado blew away their hometown. I enjoyed seeing who came to visit while I was there and meeting the siblings lined up to say good-bye.

Bobbie and Sherrie have been helping me with decorating for years. They understand my tastes and the colors I like. We move about every ten years or so (I don't know why?) and they come with fabric samples and paint colors and ladders and tools. They are so dear to me.

On one visit with this latest house I noticed they were a little down one morning. I knew they had been visiting one of their former employees who was at home dying with lung cancer. They are like that. They visit people and make them homemade coconut cream pies or, like in her case, they totally remodeled her bedroom so she could have a nice place to land in this scenario.

"Well, girls, how is Stacy doing?"

"She's terrible and sad, so sad. She's been fighting so hard for so long and it's not going to be much longer she told us. She went to see her oncologist and he told her it was time to call hospice. She doesn't want to call them. Would you go see her? We'll go with you that first time if you want," they begged in unison.

"Oh, I don't want to intrude. Let me think about this, and you make the suggestion to her and see if she's willing for me to visit. We'll go from there."

So I'm on my way home from visiting someone on Grand Lake one afternoon and get that nudge to go by and just say hi. Her home is not too far from where I was traveling.

She opened the door and acted like I there with a Publishers Clearing House check. "Hi, it's been forever since I've seen you. Did you sell that house I helped the girls paint? Come on in. My brother and his wife are here and my oldest sister."

I got to meet them and ask how she was doing. She was carrying about fifty feet of oxygen tubing around with her little tiny, four-foot frame and was wearing a Harley do rag on her bald head. The oldest sister was in the kitchen cleaning and putting groceries up and seeing what else needed to be done. But one sibling, this younger brother, was clearly having a hard time. He would go outside and smoke and then walk around and then come back in for a while. Visiting wasn't easy for him, but no one would have been able to keep him away. I also got to meet Solomon, her very dear and loyal black cocker spaniel.

He, too, was having a hard time.

I called the girls and told them I had been to visit and that I would go back in a few days. That's how we got reacquainted. I would drop by after calling and we would talk about whatever she wanted to talk about. The number one concern for her was her twin sister.

"I don't know how to help her," she said. "She's so close to me. I've always been the strongest one of the two of us. We are really bonded. How do I prepare her for my death?"

We visited about this and prayed together and Solomon lay down between us where we were sitting.

One day the girls called and said, "You might want to go see her today. Her sister called last night and she told them she's ready and to call everyone."

I was out of town that day and didn't think I would make it back the next day in time to see her. Anytime a patient who is dying tells me to call in the family, I pay attention.

But I decided to go anyway. If she had already passed, I could visit with her sweet husband who didn't say much but who loved her beyond measure.

When I drove into the yard there were several cars. I went in and all of these dear siblings were gathered around her. They had her propped up with pillows, and she was still breathing shallow breaths. They offered me a small footstool that I placed at the foot of her bed and sat down upon it. Any time I am welcomed into a setting like this, I honor and humbly realize the space is holy ground. I never take it lightly. With deep respect I bowed my head with them. Each one of these siblings took turns quietly saying good-bye and telling her how much they loved her and thanked her for all she had done for them. There were six of them. Then they began to give her permission to go on. She was in a coma-like state but not displaying any sign of pain or discomfort. Then her breathing changed and her respirations slowed and stopped.

They had all promised her they would be there and they were.

Her twin repeatedly told her, "I'll be okay. You can go. Somehow I'll be okay."

When the funeral home came to take her, Solomon followed the gurney all the way to the car.

On one of our visits she gave me a small photo of herself in a canoe on the lake behind their house. I taped it to my refrigerator. I

127

think she would like for me to remember her that way.

CHAPTER 25

HIS SWEET, WEAK SMILE

I've seen it more than once. A patient will be so near death but seemingly waiting on someone to arrive or someone to release the need to try to keep them there and then finally give them the okay. I don't know about the statistics on that or the science. I think it's all about the heart—all about the love energy that can't be measured.

I was asked to go to Sid's house to clean the deep facial wound he had from his skin cancer. This cancer had spread to his bones and his neck and his throat. But not his spirit!

He would answer the door in his pressed pajamas his sister had delivered to him regularly since he was a widower. His sister wanted to do something, anything to help.

He would whisper as loudly as he could, "Come in and let me finish this last pecan. I'm fixing you a little baggie of fresh picked out pecans that maybe you can use in a recipe for the holidays."

He didn't know that I don't cook or bake too well, so I just said thanks and was so touched that he had worked so hard on it all morning. Money can't buy gifts like this—the hours patiently and

129

lovingly devoted with these gifts of baggies holding the paper-shell–hulled pecans.

I got him into the bedroom where he had all the dressing supplies neatly laid out on the beautiful golden oak chest of drawers. He had taken his pain pill thirty minutes before as that was no easy task. But he was a brave and dear man. As gently as possible I cleaned this area and redressed it, taping it down on his fragile skin with all the precautions. Then I hooked up his tube feeding that went into his stomach, avoiding all that was wounded between lips and tummy.

He held my hands afterward and thanked me for not looking at him like he was a monster. "You, my dear man, are beautiful." He smiled a weak smile.

I had the pleasure of meeting his children who lived out of state one day. They too were so kind. He was so proud to show them off.

I got the call that he was in the hospital alone one evening and that it didn't look good. So, I decided to go sit with him a while. His daughter called while I was there, and she was so distraught that she couldn't get there before the next day. I reassured her that I would keep him company till she arrived.

But during the evening I noticed a change in his breathing. His doctor stopped by and confirmed my suspicions: his sweet little body was growing weaker and weaker. He ordered some pain medicine to be given through his stomach tube. The nurse came in and administered it within the hour. He shot me a look and gave me thumbs up that he was feeling better. He couldn't whisper anymore. He had made it plain to all of us that he didn't want any heroic measures, no more intravenous fluids, no oxygen—just pain medication as he needed it. Everyone agreed: his children, his siblings, and the medical community.

His breathing became more labored and noisy as the night wore on. I patted him hours later and asked, "Do you need more pain medicine?"

He shook his head and smiled his sweet, weak smile one more

time.

He took two more breaths and was gone.

I just sat there for a few moments holding his hand.

The nurse for his room number came in to check on him. I looked at her and said, "He's gone. You need to call his doctor and his children."

"Gone? Do you mean the gone, as in dead?"

"Yes."

"But why didn't you push the nurses' light?"

"He just passed. You walked in the room."

"But I didn't know he was going to die tonight!"

"No, we don't always know, do we? Please tell his daughter or son that I will stay here with him until the funeral home arrives. Will you close the door now?" I sat there and thanked him for the pecans again. "I appreciate getting to know you. And I'm proud to think you won't ever have to be self-conscious about your looks again." I didn't care if anyone heard me or not.

CHAPTER 26

THE BLACK SHEEP

When my supervisor asked me to go see this fellow in town I recognized his name. His last name was familiar but not the first, Samuel. "Who is this one?" I wondered.

He didn't waste any time in telling me that he was the black sheep in the family because he left after college and moved to another state and became an accountant. Everyone else in the family was a farmer or a rancher.

It was his heart. And we were to educate him about how to monitor fluid buildup and weigh every morning or report a nagging productive cough or breathing difficulty and everything else congestive heart failure can cause. We also needed to educate him on his medications and set them up for him in a pill box he would keep, he said, "in the same place all the time."

After my assessment and all that talking I needed to do, he led me into the hallway to show me the pictures of his beloved, his deceased wife, Marvene. "Look at her, nurse. Isn't she the most beautiful creature you ever saw?"

"She is."

"This one right here, this one is of her when I first met her. And this one here is of her right after we got married, but this one is after we got engaged. She was the best woman in the world, and how did I get so lucky as to find her?" Then he tenderly touched the framed photo before him.

"She told me that I should come back home if anything happened. Well, I'm here but, as good and dear as the family is, I miss her awful bad. I plan to see her again but in the mean time I've been thinking. How can I help out your business? You nurses must see so many people who don't have much. I'd like to bring a bushel of red apples down to your office tomorrow if I could and then could you take them to some of your patients?"

"Let me ask my supervisor. I'll see what she thinks and I'll call you. That's a very kind gesture," I replied.

"She'd want me to do something like this. She was always doing for others. She told me that's what we're here for. She said that if we hoard and keep all we have accumulated and never help out someone else that it's not healthy for our souls. I'm not exactly a religious man but I'd like to think I'm not a stingy one either." Then he winked.

My supervisor said she didn't see any problem with the apples but he decided to talk to his accountant and his minister and figure out a "better way" to help out others. He did.

It surprises me sometimes when I listen to a grieving spouse. It's like for the first time they are hearing what the spouse that passed said to them over the years. It's like they had filed it in a brain crevice and just now, when everyone's gone home and all of the funeral bouquets have withered, they start hearing these words bubble up from hiding.

I hope when I die my husband hears more than, "Did you get your teeth cleaned? Did you water the lawn at the office? Did you go to the dermatologist? When was your last colonoscopy?"

I've gone to so many funerals. I know that might sound morbid, but it means a great deal to a family when we honor their loved

133

one by attending the service. I find myself thinking, "What would I want to be said at my service? How will my grandsons remember me? What will my husband get up and say? What will my daughter want read? How will this affect my siblings? How do I want to be remembered?"

My patients have taught me so much.

Those who are dying and have felt the freedom to remove their masks, release their fears, make peace with their pains are the ones who really speak LIFE to me. They teach me how to live. I just need to practice it.

How do you want to live the rest of the time you have left? How do you want to be remembered?

CHAPTER 27

NO FEAR OF DYING

Frank is very up-front and honest with his declaration of "no fear of dying." And just sitting with him, at times, I find it hard to believe the diagnosis and prognosis written on his chart. Because on "good days" he's chatting and maybe able to answer the door and, perhaps, will share his World War II photo album with you.

But I have been there when the day wasn't quite as good. And on those days we might just hold each other's hands and have a little prayer per his request. But there was one especially good day and he shared stories about when he first came here to live in 1957.

"Did you know back then Ninth Street was the city limit on the south and Fifth Street was the city limit on the north?

"Did you know that back then there were no lawns that weren't mowed and there were no buildings that needed to be condemned? And there was a taxi service located south of Main Street on the west side of the highway..."

He doesn't miss a beat telling me about the service he's planning and arrangements he has made.

"I'm not afraid of dying, not one bit," he said.

"Why?" I asked with sincere curiosity.

He reared back in his recliner some and smiled and cocked his head.

"Listen and I'll tell you. Last year, I had to have some emergency surgery. I knew I was in trouble and told my wife to get me to the ER fast. Well, she did, but the doctors weren't sure I'd survive. But I didn't hear any of that. Because, all of a sudden, I was on what seemed like a huge slide in beautiful water and was heading toward the most wonderful light. There was a peace that was indescribable and no pain and no fear. Then I heard my wife say, 'Honey, don't leave me yet,' and I flipped over and headed back up the slide.

"I was in a busy ER and they were working all around me to keep me alive. Isn't that strange I wasn't hearing that entire racket? But what I did hear, clear as a bell, was her voice. And no one can tell me it wasn't real. And because of that I have hope."

I turned to his wife and asked, "Did the doctors tell you he was near death?"

"Yes," she nodded.

My friend continued. "And why I was able to come back then and now face this with perhaps only weeks...I can't answer. Maybe we needed this time we've had for some extra time to prepare? Maybe I needed some more time with my family. I don't know for sure. But what I do know for sure is that I am not afraid to die at all. Don't get me wrong. I'm not wanting to leave my wife, but when my time comes, I know I'll see that light again and I'll know that peace again. And who's to say she won't go before me or you? We just never know for sure."

It always takes me a while after a visit like this to return to laundry and cleaning house, or weeding the flower beds, coming back to Earth and reality. I can't tell you what it means to me to be allowed to visit these precious people in their space and place at the end of their lives. They bless me far more than I could ever bless them.

Occasionally, when I've had a visit like this, I go outside after dark and look up. Stars in the heavens have never failed to remind me that it's all so much bigger than I can even imagine. Stories and stars and scripture give me hope.

CHAPTER 28

NO WORDS

I heard the phone ringing and tried to sound alert when I answered it at three a.m. I was doing chaplain duty for a hospital, and the nurse wanted to know if I would come to the emergency room. A young man in his late forties had just died from injuries sustained in a car wreck. The nursing supervisor for that shift said the wife was very distraught and they weren't having any luck calming her down. She also said that she was told this woman had lost another young husband just a few years ago. When I arrived I was escorted to the chapel where the nurse was sitting with the young woman. When I was introduced to this woman, she turned on me with such anger: ranting and raving and pacing and hollering and screaming and crying. "You think you have some magic words that are going to make any difference to me? Where is your God? What have I done to deserve this? Who do you think you are coming in here and trying to comfort me?" she sobbed.

The nurse pulled me aside and told me that there was a close friend that this woman knew who lived about an hour away and would be here soon. She worked with him and she didn't want any part of me.

So I just sat there close to her and tried to "just be present." She was right. There are no words that matter much at such a time. Within a few minutes she spoke, "I'm sorry. I don't know you. It's just that I can't grasp why. And please don't say anything. That's the best part of our visit so far. You haven't tried to explain and you haven't tried to say, 'It'll be all right.' I've been through all this before just a few years ago.

"I want to scream when people tell me my husband was needed in heaven more than he was needed here. That's crap. God does not need my husband more than I do! And I'll tell you something else. I don't think he gets upset with me for being so mad right now either! Most of you minister-type people should keep your mouths shut! Let me scream. Let me cry. Let me deal with God on my terms— okay, now you can give me a hug."

I moved over and held her while she continued. Then she spoke again. "I know from experience that eventually I'll be okay again, but you have to understand that right now I'm not okay. I'm in shock and nauseated and—"

Just then her friend arrived and she rushed toward him. He held her while she cried even more. I tiptoed toward the chapel exit. He looked my way and mouthed silently, "Thank you."

I drove home and cried and prayed for her.

I felt like such a loser.

The next day I talked to my minister. He said, "It was all you could do. Grieving people teach us over and over to try to listen more and say less. When I'm asked point-blank what I think about why bad things happen like this, I don't hesitate to say, 'I don't know.' But then if they ask me if I think God was punishing their loved one or punishing them, I'm quick to say, 'No, I don't believe that.'

"This is just life with accidents, cancer, the loss of a child, so much we don't fully understand on this side.

"Our job is to listen and let them know God is okay with their anger and will be with them in their grieving process. Often it is

139

one who they know or meet who has had a similar death in their life who listens best and who understands best. They fully get how much they need their own individual responses to their loss. That lady's friend will help her. You will learn from your patients and your chaplain duty with time and experience. And, most of all, you will learn from your own loss as your life continues."

I couldn't help but think of Job when his friends came to see him.

Scripture says, "They sat on the ground with him for seven days and seven nights. No one said a word to him, because they saw how great his suffering was." (Job 2:13)

But then they messed up and tried to tell Job why they thought all his tragedy had arrived. They drove him crazy with their explanations.

I'm still learning. I try to listen more, not explain.

CHAPTER 29

INHERITANCE

I was working for a hospice agency in the '80s, assigned to help a daughter learn how to give her mother tube feedings and medications and to initiate the hospice 'talk.'"

The daughter had brought her mother to her home out in the country: a lovely place, an older but updated ranch-style home, with horses and cattle grazing on either side of the winding drive up to the house.

I had made a couple of visits to the hospital before Cecelia was discharged to introduce myself and talk about the doctor's order for her to be allowed to go home and start hospice visits. She told me then that she had agreed to the feedings to make her daughter happy, but she planned on stopping them as soon as she felt the time was right. I agreed to respect her wishes. So she greeted me with warmness like I was an old friend.

"Come in here and meet my granddaughters before they head back to college," she said. The holiday weekend was winding down and these three, stair-step, beautiful girls were all going back to the same school.

141

"Good morning, nurse. I'm the oldest. My name is Catherine. This is my middle sister, Christina, and the baby, spoiled, sister, Constance."

At that point, Constance stuck out her tongue at Catherine.

"We'll get out of here and let you talk to Grammy, and we'll return in a few minutes to see if you two need anything. Our mom has gone to town to buy a few groceries and to the pharmacy to get Grammy's meds. She should be back shortly. We're supposed to be packing. Come on, Chris; come on, Connie."

All three were blonde, but Grammy informed me that was about it as far as similarities. She said Catherine went by Cate and was focused, determined, and a caregiver of people, animals, you name it. She was a senior in her nursing program. Chris, she said, was a quieter, bookworm type from the womb. She was more of a tom-boy, and when younger loved to spend hours in their tree house with a good read. She was working on a degree in education, but was thinking about becoming a librarian. Connie, she said, was their "wild child." She didn't know what she wanted to be yet but thought she might travel the world first before she decided, and teased the family with threats of living in communes with hippies and getting a full-body tattoo.

After spending time with my patient, teaching her about her meds and pain control and comfort measures, her daughter returned and joined us. We continued to talk about hospice and then the girls came back into Grammy's room to say good-bye. I got up to leave the room and give them more privacy and my patient spoke up.

"Don't leave yet. Please finish up with my wound care while I tell these babies good-bye."

"Grammy, we'll be back home on the next holiday in four weeks. You don't have to wear yourself out now with talk," the eldest of the siblings quickly told her.

"Shhh. Sit down all three of you and, Claire [her daughter], you, too," she ordered.

And they did. All four lined up on the big western-style sofa and then clasped hands as if they knew what was coming. I was still learning and hadn't a clue!

"I know you all know this, but pretend you don't in order to spare me. I, more than likely, will not be here in four weeks. Let me finish. Claire, you have my will and know my wishes and the provisions I've made for you and Tom. Now, please fetch me my jewelry box off the bureau.

"Cate, this pearl necklace was my mother's. I want you to have it. I pray God's continued blessing on you, my dear, as you pursue your nursing career. Try not to worry so much about being a straight-A student. Learn from your patients. So much of what you need to know won't be in your books. I am so proud of you.

"Chris, I want you to have this opal ring your grandfather gave me years ago. The band on it is really worn, but you can have it reinforced if need be. You will be an excellent teacher or librarian or whatever direction you choose. You have the gift of helping children get excited about reading. You will make a difference in lives that will be remembered long after you leave this world.

"Connie, I want you to have this silver bracelet. It was my baby sister's. She's been gone thirty-some years now and she's been visiting me lately, looking just like she did when we were you girls' ages. Connie, don't let anyone dampen your enthusiasm for life. Go explore, travel, and learn well. Life will take you exactly where you need to go if you trust her. Your heart is good and, yes, we all make mistakes in our learning. But when you do, or any of you girls, admit your wrong, ask God for forgiveness and move forward.

"Don't think you were born into this family by accident. The day you were born was known by the stars long before it happened. You got purpose here, girls, so don't get lazy in living life and don't get crazy in doing too much. Find your balance, my dears. You have to make time to have fun and laugh."

They piled on her bed as tenderly as possible to prevent discomfort for her, hugging her and weeping. I was trying to turn away and couldn't see the numbers on the bag of nourishment to check how

143

much had been infused.

"Go finish packing now and then come back and kiss me bye," she told them.

Alone now, she turned to me. "You were very professional with all that. You need to know it's okay to cry sometimes in your work. You are going to see and hear and be aware of so much in this chosen career of yours. Do you realize that this is a gift from God for you to get to do this?"

I could only nod.

"Then don't be afraid. Bless people as they are, where they are."

She died before Christmas. And I wonder how those girls are doing. But, I imagine none of them has ever forgotten their grandmother's words.

I haven't.

CHAPTER 30

HOME TO BE WITH MY BOY

Mrs. Taylor's address was a rural one, and the directions were leading me deep into what seemed way too far for a mail route or school bus.

But, still, if you knew the landmarks, i.e., "the big ole' rock that looks like a feller's nose" and "you know, that red barn that used to be redder, on up the road from there past that creek with the washed-out bridge when the spring rains come..."

I carefully tackled the gate, getting the baling wire around the post like I found it after I drove through. The narrow ruts led me up to their piece of a mobile home with an added wooden addition for muddy boots.

Geese honked and hollered announcing my arrival. They scared me silly. They can bite you hard enough to draw blood. Thank goodness her oldest son came out and shooed them away.

"Outta here, you silly dang birds; let the nurse come inside."

"Sorry 'bout that, missus, but those birds think they're watch dogs. They're so good at alarming when someone pulls up, the heeler we got decided he didn't need to do that anymore. He just lies around under the porch and raises his head up to see if they need help, then falls back over. Come on in. Careful now, these cement blocks wobble a bit."

Inside in the cramped living room was my little patient. She couldn't have weighed more than eighty pounds. She was wrapped in a worn quilt with her granny glasses sliding around on her little snub of a nose.

"Come in here closer to where I can see you better. Hope you didn't have any trouble findin' us. Pull up that kitchen chair. I can't hear too good no more and I can't see none too good neither. I'm a bit of a wreck it seems. Sugar 'dibeetus' boogered me up somethin' fearful. My foot is tryin' to fall off and my heart is tired of tryin'. But doctor says he's gonna try to keep me comfortable as much as he can with sending you nurses out here to help us. Let me just tell you right off the bat I'm not takin' no more of that insulin shots and I don't give a rat's tail what my blood sugar number is. I'm done with that. I'm home to be with my boy and my little house while I can. I just want you to help me clean that foot and wrap her up and show my boy how to give me that pain medicine. We'll manage the rest all right, I guess. Decided when I got here we're gonna eat what I want to eat now."

Her "boy" turned away and walked into the kitchen and started looking in the fridge.

"I'm so proud to be home again. I got my own sheets and blankets. And my little pillow is better than that one in the hospital. Where do they buy those things? Worthless! My old cat's been laying here with me today and a couple of neighbors have been by. We got out my old spiritual records and put them on that turntable over there and listened to the Happy Goodman Family. Used to watch 'em on Sunday mornings years ago. Oral Roberts would be on a while before them. I like the old songs best.

"When you get back to that big ole' hospital, tell my doctor I'm sure proud to be home. It's like a little piece of Heaven to me before I go on to see the big Heaven. This place may not look like much to

146

anyone but me, but it's my home and it's my stuff I like, and there's so much comfort in being here. You can't put that in a pill bottle."

She fell asleep before I finished cleaning and redressing her foot. Her son told me that he was afraid to bring her home, but seeing how happy she was to be there, he was glad he did.

"I think I can give her what pills she needs when she needs them and she boasts about eating, but hasn't had a coffee cup full of anything to eat since we got here yesterday. Doctor told me not to worry about that—just let her be. He said he expects her to die in her sleep. I'm hoping."

On my way back to civilization I thought about how often we judge someone by what they look like, what they wear, or what their belongings look like.

She made me think that; perhaps, not "seeing so good" may be the best way to look at things.

She loved her little amount of stuff as much as any wealthy patient I'd seen loved their big amount of stuff. It's just all temporary stuff. Still, we like it.

CHAPTER 31

THAT 'SWEET SPOT'

One of the biggest hurdles for me as a hospice nurse was when we were trying to find that "sweet spot" where patients were not hurting and yet still able to be alert enough to talk to their family.

It wasn't always achieved.

But, with Bert, we did make it happen for a while. I don't remember exactly how old Bert was, but I do remember thinking he wasn't much older than I was, and about that time I was in my thirties. Some patients were born old, it seemed—the kind of old that carries wisdom.

He knew that he had arrived at his final battle station. So he started preparing people as best he could. I overheard so many of these conversations as I was giving him IV medications. It was almost like he would line them up, one by one, with his wife first. He talked to her about the legal papers, insurance benefits, who to call about the farm equipment, the best plumber, or when to have the oil changed on the car and he made her take notes.

Then, as I continued with his wound care, vital signs, etc., he would continue with the next person while I kept juggling how to keep him alert without him visibly showing signs of increasing discomfort. He was patient with our efforts.

His neighbor was next. "Now listen. I've been really concerned about you working so hard every day of your life. Life is short, Sam. Squeeze in a little down time."

Then more family arrived.

"Aunt Bea, you are the best cook on the whole side of my relatives. No one ever made a better peach pie. Thank you for all the cooking you've done over the years for all of us. We could taste the love in your efforts. I think you may be the best aunt ever was!"

"Son, come sit here close. Yes, you are a very young dad, but I was too. Your granddad told me a few things I'll share with you. Love those babies and your wife the very best you can. All the money in the world won't make a home. You have to learn to respect and adore Ginny, help her with baby Nate. Make one night a week a date night. Don't forget to buy her flowers every now and then or at least go out in the meadow and pick her some of those Black-eyed Susans. Tell her how much you appreciate all she does for you and your boys. They'll be grown and gone before you know it. Play ball, go fishing, attend all their sports events, know their friends and invite them over to the house so you can meet them and get to know who they're running with. Take them to church and pray with them and for them.

"Bobby Joe, thanks so much for being such a great friend all these years. No one but you would have helped me chase those dern fool cows down the drive and back toward the barn. Thanks for bringing over that cut firewood for us. I want to encourage you to get back in church. I know, I know, church sometimes is like a family...some are dear and precious and some are outright goof balls, but still they need you and your good heart."

On he would go till he finally fell asleep with no sign of pain, gently snoring. But that back screen door kept opening and closing. Some brought food, some brought flowers, and some just stood in the kitchen out of the way, holding their worn, sweat-stained western hats in their hands, not knowing what to do or say.

His wife was always grateful for any help we could give them. She told me she felt he deserved the best care and that he was a very special man. She felt honored to be his wife. She said he was always a man of integrity, always showered acquaintances with encouragement, always felt obligated to be involved in their community and church.

She told me, too, that he would wake up in the middle of the night that week and talk to her more about his love for her, saying it was a "forever love" and that it would never die, but stay alive all eternity. She said she believed him.

CHAPTER 32

THE SPIRIT OF THE HOME

A few years ago after I had retired, a friend of mine, Gina, called and asked if I could help her with her husband, Ronnie, to navigate through the hospice world. She said he had asked her to call me. They didn't "want to be a bother."

You just feel good all over walking into their home. Looks like someone would be showing up any minute to do a photo shoot for some famous magazine on style, instead of delivering oxygen.

And it wasn't just the décor, but more along the line of the *spirit* of the home. The air was full of welcome, with a "sit a while" invitation.

One of their dear, lifelong friends was in the kitchen cooking up food he might take an interest in, and cooking up food the rest of the family couldn't wait to eat. There was lots of love, even laughter, in spite of all.

After getting settled with appropriate medications, bedding, pillows, bedside table, I came to understand it was important for him to be able to see TV well to watch the Food Channel with a special fondness for Cajun food.

Over the next few days I realized cooking was only one of his passions. They had stories of famous road trips, practical jokes, the true importance of Elvis, and how proud he was when going for chemo, that the other men in the treatment room were in awe of his hair.

I learned he had an amazing power over women. There were stories about talking one woman into crawling out an upstairs window with a rope tied around her waist to help repair a leak around the chimney, a woman afraid of heights! And then he talked that same woman into posing for a photo on a bridge suspended miles above a canyon when on one of their shared road trips! She glanced at me when the story was being remembered and said, "True, every word of it, true."

Even at his weakest, he was in control. He brought his family and dear friends as calmly and as peacefully as he could to the entry of his "journey home."

He left special footprints here on earth. He was known for taking care of family and friends. He took the high road in business. He didn't worry too much about anything, trusting God with what he figured God was better at than him.

He knew about balance: work a little, laugh out loud a lot, keep good-looking hair as long as possible, avoid being stingy, play nice, honor the sacredness of love, maintain the really good friendships, and trust God with all else.

He said he thought Jesus was all about those things...except maybe not his hair.

CHAPTER 33

FEELING LIKE A MILLION BUCKS

It was so hot that summer; grasshoppers were committing suicide, throwing themselves onto the blistering pavement and looking like their own version of popcorn shrimp.

I loaded my car with sweat running down my back. Gross. I was trying to remember all Larry needed: blue pads for the bed and chair, Foley catheter, draw sheets that would enable me to turn him easier, and the patches for a bedsore that was starting to appear on his tailbone.

Walking from my car to his front steps I heard the sound of crunching gravel, but I was on grass. I let myself inside and hollered my arrival, "Larry, its meeee. I'm baaack!"

"Come on; come on in here, sis," he hollered as best he could, even though he was weak and weary these days.

"Put all that stuff down on that card table my daughter brought over here yesterday. She was tired of trying to balance everything on top of that chest of drawers. I am feeling like a million bucks, sis. I bet my blood pressure is perfect!"

I was eyeballing the urine in his urine drainage bag, which was redder than yellow and less than 100 cc.

"Now, sis, I see you're peering around to see my pee bag, but not to worry, my dear. I'm telling you, I really feel great."

I started digging out the blood pressure cuff and searching for the thermometer in his rolling bedside table when he put his cold bony black and blue hand on my forearm. "Please, sit down a minute. I'm trying to talk to you."

"Larry, what is it?" I earnestly asked while pulling up the metal folding chair the neighbor had loaned him.

He started smiling from ear to ear. "Wait till you hear this! My mother came to see me last night!"

"She did? I didn't know she was still living. My goodness, how old is the dear?" I asked in true wonder since I knew he was near eighty.

"Oh, she died years ago," he proudly announced while pulling himself up in the bed watching for my reaction.

I sat down all that I was holding and threw the blood pressure cuff on the twin bed across the room and pulled up that folding chair as close to him as I could get. I took his cold precious hand and whispered; "Tell me!" while chills were chasing each other up and down my arms and the hair on my head was on end.

"Well, it was late...way after the 10 o'clock news went off. I'd dozed off and on for a while and was trying to get comfortable when I noticed a light over in that northeast corner there," he said pointing in that direction of the room.

"Then what?" I asked getting even closer to him, not wanting to miss a word.

"Well, there she was, my mother, standing in that light, and she was smiling at me. And on either side of her were two figures in even brighter light."

"Were they angels?" I eagerly asked.

"Well, I didn't see any wings or anything like that. But they were beautiful and the whole room was full of this amazing white light and peace flooded the place, and I thought I was dying and I wasn't

154

even afraid and that's when I asked my mother, 'Mother, am I dying?' And she said, 'No, sonny boy'—that's what she called me when I was young—'I just came to tell you that you won't be alone when it's time to pass. I'll be here with you and others too. Mother loves you.'"

"Then what?" I asked in a whisper with awe and respect.

"Well, that light began to fade and she was gone. All of them were gone. But I tell you what, I believe with all my heart she was really and truly here. So, now there, you see why I feel like a million bucks today?" he asked while pulling himself up even more on his elbows.

"Yes, sir, I can only imagine. I've heard these stories before from other patients over the years. And you are one of those who, for whatever reason, got that special gift of what one patient told me was a 'glimpse of glory.'" I sighed deeply and started rubbing Udder Butter on his elbows.

"Well, I just wanted you to know, and don't tell anyone while I'm still alive. They'll think I'm crackers. I don't want anyone coming in here and trying to tell me I was hallucinating. And you don't need to keep putting that salve on my elbows or my butt!! And you can carry that new pee bag back to your car too! Don't need it either!" he beamed.

And then we both started laughing and crying and laughing some more.

When I called the next morning to get my assignments my supervisor told me not to go see Larry. He died during the night.

CHAPTER 34

ALL TALKED OUT

The directions were to go north about five miles, then west about two and a half miles and follow that gravel road into the next county. Then on the left look for a mature hickory tree with Mr. Matthews's leaning oversized mailbox next to it. Turn in there and cross over the cattle guard and drive up the winding country lane. The doublewide's at the end of the lane. "Watch your step," she said.

The few Black Angus they had were all huddled together to get under the shady trees. I looked toward the east where the creek snaked its way across their pasture. It was dry as a bone this summer.

Seemed like only yesterday it was flooded, swollen and rolling over onto the property for miles. That was just after Joe Bob's surgery, when we first met. They couldn't get the entire tumor, but did buy him some time. Same directions, same house, same patient— sort of.

I knocked gently in case he was sleeping and then went inside like she had directed me to do. "Don't expect him to be too chatty today. He's low on strength and air. But he did agree for you to show up. So good luck. I'm going to give those poor chickens some water." She turned and walked out the back utility room door and slammed the screen door they had recently added.

I made my way back to his bedroom and saw him propped up on two down feather pillows with his oxygen tubing wrapped around his ears and the prongs of the tubing in his mouth instead of his nostrils. He had his Miller Feed cap on his bald, leathery head and tipped it my direction.

"Well," I asked, "how's that working for you? Getting better air that way?"

"Yup. You don't think I'd do this for entertainment if it wasn't?" was his comeback.

He did grin, and that relaxed me completely. I sat down on the Indian blanket folded across the chair by the bed.

His whole being was gray: eyes, face, and the three hairs on his head. He looked straight at me and said, "What do you think you can do for me?"

"Well, I just wanted to see how your pain med was working and if you are comfortable and if you had any concerns or questions or requests," I said, shrugging my shoulders.

"You got all that in your black bag there?"

I started getting where he was heading. I shook my head. "No, sir."

"I'm all talked out, Becki. I'm dehydrated like my neighbor's corn crop. My skin on my forearm stands up like whipped pie meringue when I'm bored enough to check it. And, no, I do not want IV fluids.

"I'm not so much in pain as I am just restless, tired beyond any tired I've ever known, weary to the bone.

"I do not want one more well-meaning preacher to come out here and try to 'save' me. Me and God are okay.

"What question do you think I'd have at this point? I've laid here and thought about this for some time and I think I pretty well know how's this will be. It'll be a rough ride, but it won't last all that long.

157

"I appreciate you all coming out here and trying to help us though this whole ordeal since I had that first surgery. But from here on out, you can come but don't say a word. You can sit by me, but that's it. All I want from you now is to help Sue however you can. I don't know what to say to her anymore either. I never was one much with words, so I sure as hell don't know what to say to her now. Anyhow that's private."

Then he quit talking.

I just nodded and pulled the chair up a little closer.

CHAPTER 35

ALL THAT MATTERED

When I drove into his long, winding, pearl chat driveway, the multicolored leaves were chasing each other from the maples and pumpkin-colored springs of the bald cypress, too.

Canadian geese honk and holler as they make their descent in his acre-plus–sized pond.

I found myself wondering what kind of mood Tom would be in today. I took a deep breath and began mustering up courage to welcome his crankiness or his cleverness, whatever he would pitch my way.

He's admitted to me out loud, more than once, that he's not happy about "checking out" yet.

"I need more time to come to grips with this!" he said on my previous visit.

I pray while gathering my supplies to do wound care on the chest lesion from lung cancer that refused to stay in his chest.

When I knocked on the back screen door that enters into their utility room, he yells out, "Why do you always knock? Come on in!

And let the tom cat out in the process!"

His wife passed away last year, so he had been living alone until he came home from the hospital. His sister from Kansas came to stay with him until he regained some strength—or not.

I'm not too sure either one of them is tremendously fond of the other, but for now, it's working out to help keep him home.

Lou Ellen is in the kitchen making coffee and biscuits and gravy in case this is a day he'll eat a bite. She nods and offers coffee and returns to her sanctuary in the kitchen.

I approach his bed with caution. "Good morning, Tom. How's that new pain med working for you?"

"It's actually helping and I appreciate it. Taking the edge off that pain makes me less cranky. I haven't yelled at Lou Ellie [his name for her] in over an hour."

"Set your stuff down on that recliner," he continued, "and don't rush me this morning. I'm enjoying watching that foggy mist rise over the pond and listening to those geese. Did you see them landing when you were driving up?"

"Yes, as a matter of fact, I did," I answered while pulling up a chair where we could hear each other better.

The "air" is different today, and I can tell we've entered some new territory.

He eyeballs me carefully.

"What are you doing here?" he asked with all sincerity.

"What do you mean? Like my cleaning and redressing your chest wound? Or checking on your pain control? Or—"

"No. I mean what are you doing here, in life, on Earth, with your time...and your space?"

"Hold that thought. I changed my mind. I'm getting that cup of coffee. And while I'm pouring it, keep talking to me. What are you really asking me?" I said while retrieving the coffee from Lou Ellen, who was around the corner listening; she had already poured me a cup.

"Well, I've been trying to do a little introspection about how I've

160

taken up space here, how good a steward I've been with my time al-
lotment, my talents or skills, my money, and such," he answered as
he scratched his chin.

"I'm dying and I'm sorry I haven't done a better job. I let bitter-
ness set in when my wife died last year, and I've wasted good light in
a day. I could've been helping out at the church she loved so much,
or given some money to that schoolhouse where she volunteered, or
to that dang animal shelter where she carried in dog food and the
like. That's where we got ole' Tom Cat.

"And you see this all the time, and I was wondering if all you do
is work. When I was your age, I thought that was all that mattered:
make a dollar, save a dollar. Okay, that's enough. Let's get this bandage off."

And that was all he said about that ever again.

I didn't fully appreciate it. I was too busy working.

CHAPTER 36

COME SIT WITH ME

Occasionally, when my husband has had to attend a continuing education class out of state, I packed a bag and crawled in the car before he could say that I couldn't go.

This past year the class was in Albuquerque, one of my favorite places in the Southwest.

While he settles into class, I walk and read and rest and people watch, one of my hobbies. I roam all over the hotel lobby and acquaint myself with spots, like an overstuffed chair near their own Starbucks, or a designer loveseat near the concierge's desk, or a quiet corner table in the bustling restaurant.

I was on a first-name basis with as many employees of the hotel as quickly as possible. They are the real pulse of the hotel.

By the third day, I had nestled into my corner table during the post-lunch rush. I watched as she entered the dining room.

She was deliberate with her footing and handled her trustworthy cane with confidence and familiarity as she took the table next to mine.

Her attire was all at once comfortable looking and yet elegant with a color scheme that flatters her reddish-brown hair and blue-green eyes.

Her voice was smooth and deep like Maya Angelou's.

She glanced in my direction and smiled warmly, "Come, sit with me. I like to visit while I eat."

I didn't hesitate and scurried to accept her invitation, anxious to hear the story she might offer.

She was there for the nurse practitioners' conference. She had a degree in nursing, a master's in psychology, and a doctorate in education, in addition to being a nurse practitioner. Currently, she is employed by a university writing curriculum for the NP program. I was in awe.

She was curious about what I was doing in New Mexico, what I was doing with my life. She didn't waste words. I couldn't help but notice her expertise in listening.

"Hospice?" she rolled the word around in her mouth. "Hmm, tell me, have they, in your experience, ever shared with you before they pass what they are seeing?"

I nodded. "Well, yes, some do." She put down her fork and wiped her mouth with a white linen napkin.

"My sister, many years ago, had an 'experience,'" she said. "Her husband called me one night and said, 'Something's wrong with Margaret. She's in bed and she keeps passing out. What should I do?' I told him to call an ambulance and call her doctor. I met him at the ER and he told me the paramedics couldn't get an IV started in her arms and the ER team had to put an IV in her neck. I knew then she was in trouble. But in spite of nearly bleeding to death due to a ruptured tubal pregnancy, she did survive." She said that with a look of "you know what that means."

She continued. "It was weeks later when my sister and I were sitting at her kitchen table when I asked her point-blank, 'Margaret, I was wondering about your ambulance ride. Do you remember anything?' She said, 'YES!' and then she smiled.

"'What did you see?' I asked her.

163

"She leaned in and almost whispered, as if she was telling a national security secret. 'Light, such an amazing warm, beautiful light. And I heard music like you have never heard before in your life.'"

My new friend then sat up straight and pointed her fork at me.

"All this you see here right now all around us is temporary, that's all it is. There is so much we can't even begin to conceive in our wildest imaginations. We are just passing through this arena."

Was it purely accidental we got to have our visit?

I wonder.

CHAPTER 37

IN TRANSITION

Spring's winds were blowing the budding trees and flowers in Linda and Ivan's yard as if it were a choreographed dance.

They have a sign up in the entry room, advising visitors to ring the bell and come on in if you're a friend; if you're not a friend, she can still shoot her gun!

Her dear little white fluffy dog barks at my arrival, only a few barks before settling back down in his bed.

There were grandchildren visiting while on spring break and they wander through the living room where her "court" is to check on her and give her a hug or kiss.

Other family members are seeing to whatever is necessary, and the love of her life guards her nearby.

One daughter is painting her mom's nails an awesome iridescent purple color and she had matching muffins (sweater-like hand warmers) on her wrists.

She welcomes me as if I'm visiting for a planned tea party. "Come in here and sit down. I'm so glad you came by. My door is open, and I think we've had maybe 300 people here this past week. I never knew

I had so many friends," she added.

"You know, I spoke at church last Sunday. Someone from our church just happened to bring us a wheelchair, and my husband got me in it and took me to church, and I was able to get enough air in my lungs to speak and tell everyone that I'm dying and I'm ready and I want them to all be ready, too."

"I'm not afraid. I'm actually anxious for God to come get me. I've had people who visit lean over and tell me that they want me to tell their loved ones hello. I hope I can remember them all.

"Who could be more blessed than me at this stage in their life? All my children and grandchildren go to church. They all know and love God. Oh! I can't wait to see Jesus!

"I have good help with the hospice group. I love our main nurse. And, hey, look at my quilt. I've been working on this thing for years. Sew a little and put it back in the box. Get the box out and sew some more and then put it back in the box in the closet. Well, I finally got it done and I just needed to get it quilted. Our daughter took it over to that quilting place down the street and they said it'd be four to six weeks. But our daughter explained to them about my shortage of time and, look, they got it done for me and it's ready for me to pass on."

The quilt is covering her from head to toe in exquisite exotic birds of different bold colors. The quilting is beyond anything I've ever seen (I've seen a lot of quilts in my many visits to homes). What a gift!

"See, that's another God thing. Needed a wheelchair, got a wheelchair. Needed a quilt finished, got a quilt finished."

I smiled and could feel her excitement. Leaning forward I asked, "Is there anything you need?"

"No, I want for nothing. I'm just ready to go. If you do an article about me I want you to tell people they don't need to be afraid about dying. We are all in transition, that's all. We lay these clay bodies down and the real alive part of us, our spirits, move on. We go home."

166

PART THREE
FAMILY

CHAPTER 1

AFRAID NO MORE

My mother-in-law had a massive stroke in the early '80s. A friend of hers noticed at the convenience store she owned that when she arrived to open the front door early that morning that she wasn't speaking clearly and thought I should come get her to take her to the hospital. When I arrived I could see that she was in distress and headed as fast as I could to the hospital ER. Her blood pressure was extremely high and as they attempted to bring it down, it only went higher. She was flown on a medical helicopter with me by her side to the big city hospital where the stroke continued, it left her paralyzed on her right side and without her speech. The look in her eyes was pure fear.

After weeks of rehab she learned how to help herself by using a cane with "feet" and how to dress herself and perform the activities of daily living with minimal assistance. Finally, there was some return of speech, and she came home. I still remember her smile that night as we tucked her into her own bed and watched her drift off to sleep.

She was able to live at home for a few years with occasional help from the Home Health Agency and family, but then she fell in her bathroom one day and broke her hip and her arm. After surgery and recovery we took her to a local nursing home for extended rehab and strength rebuilding so she would be able to return home, but she was there for twelve years due to several more small strokes.

During that twelfth year, after an exam by her doctor due to her complaint of abdominal discomfort, she was scheduled for x-rays and then surgery because of a partial bowel obstruction. Even though she understood it was risky she wanted to proceed. She said she didn't want to die, and was afraid it might be cancer and wanted to get rid of it.

A couple of weeks after she returned to the nursing home, she called me wanting to talk to her son. I explained that he was out of town on business and asked her if I could do anything for her. She said she needed to talk to me in private. So I went to her room and sat on the edge of her recliner and said, "What's going on?"

She said, "Close my door first."

I got up and closed the door and focused all my attention on her. She began.

"I died while I was in the hospital," she said, smiling like it was really good news.

I had heard enough by then from my patients to not take this lightly. "What happened?" I asked while I placed my hand on her arm.

"I was in the operating room and all of a sudden I was above my body and I heard the doctor say, 'We're losing her! We're losing her!' And then I floated up higher into the corner of that room and I could see all the instruments and all of the nurses rushing around and I felt fine. I didn't have any pain."

"Did anything else happen?"

"Yes," she nodded and smiled again. "I saw some of my family. The thing I wanted you all to know is that I am not afraid to die anymore."

Years later we received a call one night while out to dinner that she was in the ER in respiratory distress and didn't look good. We drove to the hospital. When we got into the room she was in the nurse said they needed to intubate her and put her on a respirator. Even in her distress she was alert enough to hear that and raised her hand, shaking her forefinger back and forth. I bent over and said, "Do you want the respirator?" She shook her head, no.

The doctor stepped closer and said, "What can we do for all of you?" We asked for a private room, oxygen if she wanted it, medications to assist in less respiratory discomfort if needed and paperwork to sign for a "Do Not Resuscitate" order. She nodded.

We moved to a private room and settled in with her. I asked her if she was afraid. She shook her head no. And she weakly smiled. We elevated her head and talked to her to reassure her that we would stay with her. She denied pain and she began sleeping. Her son and two daughters all spoke with her and showed her their love. We all spent the night as she grew weaker and moved into a semi-comatose state. Early the next morning her breathing changed and she peacefully, quietly quit breathing.

I've heard stories like this many times in my career. I never tell a patient that they are hallucinating or dreaming. I listen.

CHAPTER 2

POSITIVE ATTITUDE EQUALS POSITIVE MEDICINE

Aunt Chris is married to our dad's twin brother. I met her when I was about three or four years old when my mom married our step-dad. I remember thinking she was so pretty and nice. As we grew up over the years she always remembered all four of us kids at birthdays and Christmases. She would sing us songs, paint our nails, tell us stories, and made everyone of her nieces and nephews on both sides of the family feel like that they were the most important people.

She prayed about everyone's needs, ailments, and fears. She loves all of life. And she trusts God with all things. So, when she called to let me know a few years ago about her breast cancer diagnosis, I think my heart stopped for a few moments. "Not Aunt Chris!" But then I took a deep breath and said, "May I go with you to your first chemo after surgery?"

"Yes, I want you there since you worked in oncology before. Your uncle is not too good at sitting still and I need a calming presence. So right after surgery she was sitting up in bed and blessing everyone who came in to see her. She cheered the nurses and doctors, the housekeeping staff and visitors. In record time she was healing and eager to start chemo. She wanted to know everything there was to know about the pre-meds and the chemo meds, the side effects of radiation, and what she could do for herself as far as nutrition, among other things. But also very important to her was her circle of family and friends praying. She blessed the oncologist; she blessed the chemo nurses and everyone who visited. She did well, very well.

A few years after that she was told by her heart doctors that she needed to have heart valve replacement. The tricky part of this, the surgeon said, was that her skin on her chest was fragile due to the radiation years before. But being very brave again she went into surgery with a very positive attitude and cheering all the family on, instead of being the one in need of cheering. After the surgeon came out and said all went well, we waited for her arrival back to her room, a special ICU/family/waiting room in a heart hospital. She didn't want to wake up for some time. One of the nurses decided she needed to wake up so he leaned over and said very loudly, "CHRIS! OPEN YOUR EYES!"

She jumped straight up in the bed and scared that poor boy half to death. All her tubes were jiggling and my two sisters and I jumped off the visitors' couch. We didn't know whether to punch him or sit back down at first.

Hours later I felt like it was okay to go down the street and eat some dinner. Within minutes after ordering I got a call from my cousin that they were rushing my aunt back into surgery due to a tear in one of the arteries and a gross amount of bleeding. They couldn't assure us that she would survive. All kinds of prayer began around that crowded waiting room. And within an hour the surgeon came out and said, "Folks, she's stable. We were able to repair that artery and she has quit bleeding. We believe she's had a miracle tonight." I still get chills when I write about this so many years later.

A few years, after that ordeal, she was diagnosed with a second breast cancer. How can one person have so many serious diagnoses?

But, once again, with faith and her sweet spirit, she went for surgery and had her second mastectomy. Again she was very brave and positive and trusting God. She told all us, "Now listen, I'm going to be fine." Then she was told by her primary physician that she needed to have her thyroid removed. Her motto remained: "Trust God, pray believing, bless and encourage others!" She sailed right through that one too. Recently she was diagnosed with diabetes. She got proactive again and started reading all she could on diabetes and how to manage her diet, medication, and lifestyle. Then, lo and behold, my uncle was diagnosed with diabetes. She helped educate him as well.

Why do some people fare so well with so many challenges and some faint and fall over with the common cold? Is that because of what we grew up with? Is it because of our own spiritual growth pattern in life? Is it a choice?

One patient told me, "Listen, I can choose to be positive or negative. I can choose to read positive or negative stories. I can listen to music or TV that's positive or negative. I don't care who your people are. I get to choose if my glass is half full or half empty no matter what my DNA says!"

I think my aunt makes that choice every day, several times a day!

CHAPTER 3

A CONTINUED STORY OF GOOD-BYES

It was a long trip to Indiana that first time after I got the call that my biological dad had been diagnosed with cancer. John drove me up there while I dealt with all those childhood memories forcing their way out of hiding.

He and my mom divorced when I was three. So when he came for visits to Oklahoma I was so excited to see him and then horrified when he had to leave. Poor man. I would cling to his neck as they separated us for him to leave. When I got older I would ride on a Greyhound bus to the Hoosier State to spend a few days and then crawl back on when it was time to go. I cried while crossing at least two states before falling asleep.

He loved me more than anyone had ever seemed to love me as a child. He looked at me knowing I was underweight, had buck teeth, long skinny feet, and none-too-exciting brown hair. He still seemed proud that I was his daughter.

He had a stroke that left him without much speech a few years before, so as I sat with him on his cement steps out on the front porch he was hesitating in his words. The doctors had been plain in speaking the truth about his tumor. Surgery would not do any good and any treatments wouldn't either. He had maybe a couple of months, maybe weeks to get his things in order. His wife had made me promise not to cry. I was choking to death trying. "Becki, love you always. Hurt bad in hip and chest. Not bury in Oklahoma, okay not to be in place with my parents. Bury here in Indiana. Me and God good."

In my mind, I was three again and he was being torn away from me. But I had promised, so I smiled the best I could and just nodded in agreement and understanding of his requests.

We drove home with me sobbing for many miles. And then there was the not knowing when to return "in time." I talked to them every other day or so and tried to figure this out. Experience with my patients had told me over and over that there are no ways to be absolutely sure of the day. So with many prayers asking God when to pack my bag to fly back north, I left one day unsure of when I would return.

Within two days of my arrival he was hospitalized and put on a morphine drip to help control the awful pain. I didn't leave his bedside for those last five days. I would try to use all my experience; it didn't help much. I did know how to monitor his pain relief, but I was his child, not his nurse. The more he started fading, the closer I got to him. I held his huge, brown hands and memorizing the lines in them and the smell of them. Finally, I let the bedrail down and crawled up in the bed next to him and cradled him whispering, "Dad, Dad...can you hear me? I love you so much, and I want you to know that I got this big ole' heart from you. I love animals like you do. I love people like you do. I know you are hurting and you need to know it's okay to go on. I will miss you like crazy, but I will be okay."

He sighed deeply, but was already in a coma. I knew he had heard me. He died quietly the next day. It sure felt like part of me went with him.

I try to remember this when I'm sitting with someone. A child is a child all of his or her life. I don't care how old you get. Losing a parent is huge. Have mercy on anyone you know who comes upon that first Father's Day or Mother's Day without a beloved parent.

CHAPTER 4

AS MEAN AS A SNAKE?

They always said Aunt Vera was as mean as a snake. They told us kids not to rile her when we went to visit. So I made the drive to their home with mixed emotions to see my uncle who was dying with heart disease. I was sure hoping that she was not upset about anything while I was there.

She wasn't. With the exception of not being able to do much for my uncle, she was pretty calm and, as always, in control. She watched those hired caregivers with an eagle's eye, making sure no one mistreated him. They had no idea of the hell to pay if they had!

She had been through a lot herself the past few years with bilateral mastectomies and the worst case of shingles I had ever seen or heard tell of. She didn't flinch one bit. She did what had to be done and got on with business.

He took good care of her and she was "by damn" going to see about him all the way.

I wondered sometimes why she was as angry as she was. The older I got the more I figured out that most folks have a reason for being so mad for so long. I heard that she had a father who was pretty rough on his fourteen kids; she was the baby.

My aunt and uncle owned a bar they opened back in the late '30s or early '40s. She was respected all over the county. It was the poor fool from out of town who came in thinking he could smart off at her, or the crazy fool who once thought he would try to rob her. She took a pool stick to him. I think I heard he moved out of state. No one ever tried anything so silly ever again. She had put her shotgun up on the bar every few days or so for a couple of minutes while getting someone a pickled egg out of a gallon-sized jar. It was a peaceful place.

We grew up going there to visit, and I loved sitting on the footrest of that long, beautiful mahogany bar. I would watch people come in and play shuffleboard, and I would watch my aunt throw some kind of red, oily, sawdust-looking stuff on the floor and then get out a long mop-like broom and sweep that red stuff up. It smelled good. I can remember it still.

When I was very young I went out to the minnow tanks they had south of the bar. I guess I fell in because my mom said that when they found me I was hanging on by my fingertips.

All these memories are roaming around in my mind while I go to see them. They didn't want to sell the bar, but a new highway was coming through and they wanted to come through my aunt and uncle's bar, The Red Heart Inn. So, with a nice chunk of change they moved and began a new life after building a home that sat upon a hill not too far away. She hated it. He loved it.

She was sitting on the couch not too far from his hospital bed watching him and trying to breathe herself with coiled oxygen tubing next to her. When I approached her she said, "I'm glad you are here. Your sister is on her way."

My uncle barely fit on the bed being so very tall. He gave me the sweetest smile and a faint "Good morning, Becki." I leaned over and kissed him gently on his bald head. I took my stethoscope out of my bag and began listening to his heart. His heart rate was so very irregular and weak. He glanced at me and winked. With as much

179

professional attitude as I could muster, I continued to assess him. The urinary output was poor, his appetite next to none, his fluid intake poor as well. His spirit was strong, though.

She got up and came to his side and he smiled even broader. She leaned as close as she could and said, "Ude, you all right?" And when he nodded, she returned slowly and with caution to the couch.

I called my supervisor and told her that my uncle's status was very poor and requested that I might stay with them. I pulled one of the dining room chairs close, put my hand through the rails of the bed, and held one of his hands. He closed his eyes and slept with a soft little snoring that gave my aunt permission to close her eyes as well.

As I returned to the dining room table to chart, I heard him whispering and thought he might be dreaming. I tiptoed close and heard him clearly praying.

"Please, God, have mercy on her. Forgive her in Your grace the way You have forgiven me. Please, God, have mercy on my wife. I don't know if she's asked you yet or not and I want to ask for her. Thank you. Amen."

I couldn't move quickly enough away to the darkened narrow hallway and held my weeping in my hands. My heart was so full of love and awe for him hearing how much he loved her even now.

CHAPTER 5

LITTLE SISTER

Cindy is not very tall but, boy howdy, she is strong and can work circles around me. I watch her sometimes while showing up unexpectedly for a visit. She's running the vacuum, which I'm sure outweighs her, dusting and mopping and fixing a three-course dinner from scratch. If she took a tiny break, she would watch a little bit of an old movie she had recorded. And, if she had time, she would get on the mower and mows a couple of acres.

Her cherub face was beet red and her Tinkerbelle-sized feet might have been swelling a little bit. She didn't complain.

She loves retirement and all the chores of gardening, harvesting, and then canning, freezing, and Lord, if the grandkids come over, she plays games with them and fixing them treats.

Once, she showed me the insides of her refrigerator (I think the contents are alphabetized) and freezer where she had prepared a week's worth of dinners. My husband says I didn't get that gene.

She saves coupons, fixes meals for her church, and helps them sew aprons for nursing home patients' walkers to put their remotes or phones in while they walk around. (I didn't get that gene either! I couldn't sew two dishcloths together and make a decent tea towel.)

I knew her when she was little and she was like this then too. She would save every penny; she saved her Halloween candy for weeks. She cut her own hair and was really disappointed the first time she cut her Barbie's hair and it didn't grow back.

She married a guy I was kind of wary of when I first met him and I told my husband he needed to find out what his intentions were and if he was okay. He was. He cracks me up now when I see them together and he's grinning at her watching her do another good deed.

She's had some health issues over the past few years that have been scary for us to watch. But she has taught all of us to relax and not worry so much. She said that she was not going to any more hospitals and would haunt anyone who puts her in another ambulance.

She also told us that she was going to continue doing what she does every day and trust God with her "timing."

Honestly, I don't remember anything she has ever done to hurt, offend, or upset anyone. She doesn't gossip, drink, chew, cuss, or anything like that. Those were some of the things our grandma said were signs of backsliding. And, even though she is younger than me, she has taught me a lot about faith.

Even though she cans and freezes those garden pickings for the future, she is living it all day by day.

CHAPTER 6

I MADE IT! I MADE IT!

My husband's sisters both telephoned us, first one and then the other. "Would you two please go see Uncle Fred and check on him? His wife's brain tumor has grown so much that their doctor has called in hospice, and they don't think she has long.

My husband does not like hospitals, "death beds," or nursing homes, but he said, "We need to do this."

We were taking our grandson to college and had a caravan of supporters with us ushering this child into his freshman year and away from all of us. He was excited and our daughter was trying not to cry all day. His friends were giddy with joy of all the new freedoms they were getting ready to experience. So, by the end of a very long day, we didn't know if we had enough emotional strength to go see Uncle Fred and his sweet wife.

But we went. And we met her family for the first time and visited with Uncle Fred about how she was doing. He has always been a matter of fact kind of guy and said, "Well, she doesn't have long. We got her in a hospital bed next to mine. She's not talking as much but she is still talking a little every now and then. She still knows me and her family. Let's go on in there and you can tell her you're here."

We tiptoed into the room and respectfully approached her bed. Her face was still and, even that day, so beautiful. Her white hair graced her face and she had a soft, pretty gown on and nice comfortable bedding. Can she really be that close, I wondered?

I bent down and whispered her name. She smiled without opening her eyes. I told her who I was and that we were praying for her. I also told her that we had met all of her lovely family. She turned her head slightly toward me and acknowledged she knew me and my husband who then came closer and took her hand and expressed his caring thoughts as well. When he backed away I bent near her right ear and whispered, "I'm praying that you know God's abundant love for you and that you know you will not make this transition alone. Your angels and your family and others who've gone before you will come. I'm praying for you to know glimpses of glory in your sleep tonight so you can see where you are heading and have great peace and assurance."

She opened her eyes and turned her head toward me. "Becki, please keep praying for me. Thank you for sharing that." And she turned toward the wall and closed her eyes and didn't respond anymore. We tiptoed out.

Within a couple of days we received the call that she had passed away. I was thankful for her but sad for my husband's uncle, her family, and her friends. This was his second wife to die. I was unable to attend the funeral as I was heading to a writing retreat. My husband called me and told me that his uncle was doing as well as could be expected and that he was again in the "matter-of-fact" mode. His uncle told him that the Holy Spirit had carried her home and now he would try to start another new life.

Two days after arriving in Sedona, Arizona, I went to see a spiritual counselor I see every year there. We talk about spiritual growth and our journeys here.

"Before we begin, I want to tell you that I sense a very strong presence of someone older, maybe in her eighties, with white hair, and she's insistent that I tell you how much she appreciates you helping her in her transition. Do you know who I'm seeing?" she asked.

"No, I've been doing that for thirty years. It could be so many different women."

"No, this lady is saying you helped her recently. You talked to her about being okay with her leaving here and moving forward. "

I slapped my face with both hands and exclaimed, "Oh, my. I know who this is. We just visited her last week. Her funeral was two days ago."

My friend was smiling and said, "That's it! She's jumping up and down and saying, 'Tell them all at home that I made it!! I made it!!'"

There again, when someone shares something like that with me, I don't try to tell them they're crazy. I listened and I thanked God and my husband's uncle's wife.

CHAPTER 7

MY MOM

We knew Mom was not as mentally strong as she had been in younger years. And for about the past ten years she would surprise us on occasion with a big forgetful moment, like the time our daughter called and said, "Mom! Granny Mary was in the same store as me just now and I saw her and I said, 'Hi, Granny, what are you doing here?' And she said, 'I have four children and their names are Becki, Patti, Cindy, and Jeffrey.' And then she turned around and left. What's wrong with her? Do I need to call someone about taking her home? Is her husband strong enough to come get her? She scares me when she talks like that!'"

I told her not to follow her. She goes to that store every day and walks back to her house, her husband told me. I told her that if she approached her she might get agitated and deck her. She had been known to do that in the past if provoked.

So, when the police from her town called me that Sunday night, I wasn't exactly surprised. "Ma'am, your mother keeps calling us at the police station and saying someone's out to get her and they want to kill her. We've been out there to her home four times this week-

186

end and we can't see anything suspicious. Her husband said she's okay, but he didn't look too okay either. We thought you might want to know and get her some medical attention. She gave us your number."

I called her husband and asked him if I could come get her in the morning and take her to the doctor or a hospital. He agreed and said he would keep her in the house.

When I arrived and explained to her that the nice policeman called me and that we were going to see the doctor because he said they couldn't come back to check on her until she went, she agreed.

"They are whispering and I can hear them in those floor vents. Oh, you have to be careful too because they heard me giving the policeman your phone number!" She exclaimed with wide open eyes.

And, I swear to God, for a few seconds I thought, "Oh, shoot!"

We drove to the nearest mental hospital and went in to see if I could get her examined or admitted for observation. Nope. They were full. So then I told them what she told me on our way inside. "Becki, I need you to take me to the pawn shop so I can buy a pistol. I need to be able to protect myself."

"Oh, well, maybe you could see if her doctor would see her today and make a suggestion."

I got her back in the car and called a good friend at my local hospital where I knew people. She told me to drive back there and let them examine her in the ER to see if she's having some difficulty with a stroke or a clogged artery and we could go from there.

She chatted all the way to the hospital, all happy about us spending some quality time together. I felt ashamed. I was always busy seeing other people and not visiting her enough.

She had the ER doctor, God love him, laughing with nearly every serious question he had asked her. "Mrs. J., could you tell me who the last president was?"

"Hell no! I'm not political. They ought to fire all those SOBs in Washington!" and then she would laugh.

"Okay. Can you count backwards in tens for me?"

"Are you kidding me? [She really said another word!] Don't you have a calculator or something to figure that out with?"

"Okay. Do you know what year it is?"

"Okay, you're starting to piss me off here, doc. I've been having serious problems with crazy people wanting to kill me because I smoke cigarettes. They are talking loud enough from their condo; I can hear them in our vents. And you want to know what year it is? I'm getting out of here if you can't get me a cup of coffee. No, better than that, let my daughter take me outside that ER door and smoke me a cigarette. You people are starting to make ME crazy!"

With that the ER doctor, God bless him again, said she needed to be evaluated at the Alzheimer's unit in the town west of there, and he would make a call.

I felt so much relief that we were finally going to get some help for her. I was happy to take her outside for a smoke. She was talking to a real live beetle one moment and laughing about the crazy doctor the next. I could feel my neck and shoulder and back muscles tying up in major knots.

The ER doctor came to get me and told me they couldn't see her until Wednesday and they could admit her then. He said to take her back to her husband and where she has familiar surroundings. Then he said to take her to the other hospital on Wednesday morning at nine.

I did.

That interview for admission was similar to the ER visit. But then the unthinkable. This well-meaning admission employee asked her, "Ma'am, have you ever considered suicide?" I quit breathing.

My poor tough mom looked at her lap and started crying while answering her and watching me. "When all my kids were very young, about ages one through six, we ran out of food. My husband's job was over and we didn't want to ask anyone for help. I remember thinking that if I killed myself someone would help them. Then I prayed to God for help and a relative drove up and brought us some groceries and some cash and said not to tell anyone. I've never thought about it since. Someone told me you can't go to Heaven if you kill yourself and I've never wanted since then for any one of my kids to find me if I did."

The lady said she would be right back. We were led into the unit behind closed doors and into a nice room. They told us her doctor would see her later. Mom said, "Well, I'm sure as hell glad they lock those doors so those crazy people who are after me can't get in."

She liked her room and she asked me to go to Wal-mart and get her some cigarettes, some Certs breath mints, and a paperback novel. She always did love to read.

It was close to Mother's Day so I bought her a new pair of walking shoes as well. She was walking six miles a day before I picked her up two days before. I thought she would like to walk again when she was able to go home.

She settled in fairly well and was taking her medications. Then all four of us kids were planning on coming to see her on Saturday for a great family visit.

Thursday she wanted to go back home and get her husband to come live with her there. She was eating and sleeping well, they said. I visited during visiting hours after two p.m.

Friday she wasn't exactly thrilled to be there but wanted to "jump through all the hoops" to get the policeman to come back to check out those crazy people who were threatening her. And she wasn't eating as well. But her husband did come to visit; that made her happy.

On Saturday I called the ward and asked to speak to her nurse. It was about eight a.m. I wanted to know how she was doing. "Well, she doesn't want to get up and eat her breakfast."

"That's not like her! She loves to eat, and she gets up early every morning of her life! I want to visit and talk to her." I gasped and trying to remain calm.

"You can't do that. Visiting hours start at two and they don't make exceptions. Come at two," she flatly announced.

"Okay, but if anything changes, you call me right away! Tell her I

189

said to get up and get dressed because all her kids are coming to visit today at two p.m. and maybe that will help."

Within twenty minutes they called back, "You need to get here as fast as you can."

I threw the phone down and drove over the speed limit the ten minutes it took to get there—like a woman possessed. But I knew. I knew.

When I entered the area they stopped me at her door and said, "Wait. The doctor wants to talk to you."

I said as nicely as I could, "You move away from that door. I am a hospice nurse, and I've been with many people who have died. I want to be with my mother!"

She did.

The code blue team was cleaning up. Mom was lying there still, white, gone. The doctor said, "Everyone, let's let her be with her mother. Mrs. Hawkins, I will be outside if you want to talk to me." I waved them away.

I went to her and sat with her and said, "Mom. I know you might still be here waiting on me, so I just want to tell you it's all right to go. Go to your parents and your siblings and your first baby and all those angels and all the healing and light and love you'll know now forever. We'll be okay. I'll look after the others. You're free now, Mom. I love you."

Then I walked out the room and down the hall to the nurses' station. "How can we help you, Mrs. Hawkins?"

"Would you please allow me to use a private room with a phone so I may call my siblings who are on their way here to visit her? I also need to call her husband."

And that's what I did.

Sometimes families or spouses left behind will tell me of having conflicting feelings of relief that their loved one isn't suffering anymore and guilt for feeling the relief. Me too. Even though it's sad to say, I was just so angry for so long at those employees at that hospital, even though they were just following orders. I had been with so many patients who had died and tried to give them and their families the best I knew to give. I felt robbed of getting to be with my mother. It took me years to begin to think that perhaps it was just meant to be that way. What I do believe now, more than ever, is that ALL IS WELL and that there is purpose in all things, even if they seem insane and beyond explanation. Scripture says that right now we see in the "mirror" dimly, kind of like a cloud and that one day we will see clearly. I have to trust that. We can trust God with all of it. I don't have to feel that guilt anymore. I don't have to question myself, "Why didn't you force your way into that hospital ward!?"

I have peace now. But I don't try to shove my convictions on anyone else: family, friend, patient, or patient's family. I try to just be present and listen without judgment or criticism or any finding of fault. It's an imperfect world here. We have to take care of each other, love one another. I don't think Christ was joking about that.

CHAPTER 8

MY BROTHER'S KEEPER

My brother Jeffrey was the youngest of four siblings and I was the oldest. I'm not exactly sure how Jeffrey and I became so connected, but I do remember Mom making me sit with him on the couch after school when he was in the first grade to help him learn to read. I felt like, "Why me!" And I also felt like, "I better do this so he doesn't get yelled at."

I also remember all four of us hiding in our parents' closet one night when they were out. We didn't have locks on our door. We had heard a noise outside so I herded everyone into the closet. I took the butcher knife with me. Then, for some reason, I began to giggle. My younger sister looked at me and quietly said, "If you don't stop laughing, I'm going to take that knife away from you and cut your throat." I started laughing out loud! I could see Jeffrey looking at me as though he wasn't sure if he was supposed to be scared anymore.

I was the first to leave home at age eighteen. The only good thing about that for Jeffrey was that he finally got a bedroom to himself. For some reason he and Dad didn't see eye to eye very often. But

Mom adored him and tried to protect him.

I was so busy being a new wife and then a new mother and working at a full-time job that I wasn't around enough during those very crucial years of twelve to eighteen when he was still at home. But when I did visit he would stand in the gravel driveway and say, "Peel out, Becki, peel out!" as I was leaving. So I would peel out just for him, making my tires spin as fast as I could. Then he would pretend his bare feet were tires and run down the road "peeling out" and making tire squealing noises.

His teenage years were very troublesome. He didn't like school, he hated living at home, and he wrecked three cars, a pickup, and two motorcycles. It really was a miracle he had survived any of those accidents. During those years he was introduced to alcohol, marijuana, and hard drugs. And he liked the escape they gave him. How on earth he lived long enough to graduate from high school is still a mystery to me. I pulled out some old photos recently and one was of all four of us at our grandparents' home the winter before he graduated. We girls were all smiling; he wasn't. The last few years I've dreamt of being back home as a teenager and trying to make my parents happy and somehow save my brother from unhappiness.

All of this is swirling around in my thoughts as I wait for him to come out of his radiation treatment each of those thirty-three days. I'm tormented with the thoughts, "I'm guilty; I could have saved him, and I should have rescued him from those choices he made." They are ridiculous thoughts—I know that—but they are bubbling up from somewhere deep inside me. "Maybe if he'd been happier he wouldn't have smoked all those cigarettes!" Again, stupid thoughts. Would I feel the same way if it had been skin cancer instead of lung cancer?

I recalled how years before he had been arrested because of too many DWI tickets. His attorney called me and said he might be able to get him into a drug and alcohol rehab and prevent him going to prison. I didn't have much hope, but I sure didn't want him incarcerated. How would that help?

Then one day after he had been in the rehab for weeks, his nurse called me. "We are not supposed to let our clients talk to anyone from home while they are here, but your brother is suicidal and he wants to talk to you. Will you speak to him?"

"Yes, of course!" I said all the while thinking, "What am I going to say that could help?" He came on the line and told me he didn't think he could go on anymore due to the emotional pain he was working on getting up and getting out and trying to heal. "I don't think I can keep this up."

I was stifling sobs but replied forcefully, "Listen to me. I know you can do this. Look at all you have survived. You can survive this, too. This is your chance to have a new life and a good life. I believe in you and I'm praying for you and so are all the rest of the family. We all love you. Do not give up. You are stronger than you think!"

Then the nurse took the phone from him and thanked me and hung up. I slid down the wall to the floor and wept until I could not anymore. He did make it. And he was sent to a halfway house in a town about ninety minutes away from us. The attorney called and said we needed to go to court to see if the judge was going to let him stay in the halfway house or go to prison.

His attorney asked me to appear in court and to testify about why I believed that Jeffrey should be allowed to continue "working the program" and living in the halfway house instead of going to prison. I told the judge that before he went to rehab I didn't know if he would ever be able to stay out of jail, but after rehab he was a new man and I believed I had a brother who now had another chance at life.

So that judge sternly warned Jeffrey than if he was arrested one more time he would go to jail. He allowed him to return to his halfway house. Even though he was on probation, he gratefully headed back to his new home.

One day he called to see if I would like to visit and go to an AA meeting with him. I did. When he spoke that day my chest filled up with so much pride, joy, and thanksgiving that I thought I would burst into a million little pieces.

He was a welder and worked in that town honing his skills making new AA friends and friends in the community. He was doing some heat and air conditioning work and some tile work and some construction and everyday—and everyday going to an AA meeting. When his probation was over he decided to weld full-time for a company in his new town. When they tested him they saw how really good he was at the art of welding. They hired him on the spot. He did this for years until another friend called and asked him to start welding along the U.S. coastlines for an oil company. He took the job. So every week he would call home and tell us where he was, what he was doing, what sight-seeing he had done, how the local AA group was, and all he was learning.

He was reading again, he told me. Suddenly I was in a flashback to a couch in our childhood, and in my mind I turned to him and rubbed his burr-cut head of hair, remembering Dick and Jane and Spot and Puff from his first grade reading book.

During this time of traveling he was feeling really weak and decided to go to a doctor. After his exam and some lab work the doctor called him a few days later and told him he had Hepatitis B and C. What a blow! He asked me to go see the specialist with him not too far from our home. The specialist's nurse taught him how to give himself the injections to fight the hepatitis and when to go for lab work to check his blood cell counts that might get too low with this medicine. He didn't flinch. He educated himself about the drug, the side effects, the disease process, the blood work, and gave himself all of the injections that the doctors prescribed to him. He said he ached and had extreme fatigue; he felt depressed and mad. He said he wasn't sure how he had contracted the disease but suspected from his older tattoos or hard drugs with bad needles before he got clean and sober. By then it didn't matter. He kept losing weight, and I didn't know if he would survive this or not. But he did finish the injections prescribed and the lab work, which showed that his liver was getting better. The doctor said he couldn't use the word "healed," though.

He continued working along the coasts. When he would come home he would occasionally speak to an AA group somewhere in the state or his local area or even at the local high school to a group of teens about the dangers of drugs and alcohol. Dad was pleased. And in their own ways, a road to some peace and forgiveness and healing was being paved due to Jeffrey's education in AA and a boatload of prayer from family and friends.

He came home for her funeral when Dad's second wife passed away. Dad asked him if he would be interested in having the home place when Dad passed. My brother said he would really like living at the home place again someday. Within a few months Jeffrey called Dad and said he was really tired of traveling and wanted to know if he could come home and live with him and find a job locally. He was tired in many ways. Dad and his little dog were lonesome. Another person around the house to talk to and argue with and discuss the upcoming winter weather sounded like a good idea. He found a job and got acquainted with the local AA group. We had a year of what some refer to as normal.

A year later I ran into him at Wal-mart and he said, "Hey, I was getting ready to call you. The doctor wants me to have a CT scan of my lungs this coming Monday. I've been coughing more than usual, and the antibiotic he gave me didn't do much good. And I've been coughing up some blood. Do you think you could meet me there and go through all that rig-a-ma-roll paperwork they ask for?"

"Sure, I'll be there." I said. As he walked away I realized I was trembling. He was thinner and his color was abnormal.

When Monday arrived I wasn't prepared for what he looked like. He was pasty pale and he couldn't move his left arm in a full range of motion. He was nearly in tears with fear and coughing up more blood.

I summoned from the depths of my courage and said, "Hey, let's get in there and get this test done. Maybe it's a pinched nerve. We'll see about some radiation to help if it's something different. We'll find out what's going on and then we'll make a plan. Don't worry, I'm going to help you every step of the way."

His doctor asked us to pick up the CT scan results and said that he had made an appointment with a lung specialist in two days.

I read the printed report. It wasn't good.

My brother and I, my little sister and her husband, Dad and his twin brother all went for the appointment. She gave us the clear picture, showing us in color the tumor and where it was in the lung. It was wrapped around his aorta.

She made an appointment with the hospital for a bronchoscope to get a biopsy of the lung tissue with the tumor to see what we were dealing with so we would know how to move forward.

It was an aggressive lung cancer. She told us that there wasn't a cure but they might be able to slow it down with chemo and radiation. She contacted an oncologist for us. They would see us in twelve days. That seemed like too long to both of us.

A few days later we went to our other sister's birthday party about ninety minutes away. He wanted to be there for her and to see everyone. All the family was there so that made it nice. But on the way home he was not feeling well; he was chilled and coughing. When we arrived home I asked him if I could take him to the ER. He decided he wanted to see if he might feel better after he got in his recliner and took some Advil. He promised he would call if he started feeling any worse.

I went home and was just about asleep when the phone rang. All I could hear was him choking. I told him I was on my way. I called Dad, who was in his bedroom and oblivious to Jeffrey's choking, and told him to rush in there, sit him up, shake him, and see if he was okay. I called 9-1-1.

When I arrived the ambulance was there and Jeffrey was being put on a gurney. He was blue. He was taken to the local hospital. The chest x-ray revealed pneumonia in addition to the tumor. He was started on IV antibiotics and then one of the doctors came in and talked to me about getting him to the larger hospital "RIGHT

AWAY" where the lung specialist and oncologist were. The problem was that the ambulance wouldn't be available for hours. I loaded him in my car, IV and all, plus the x-ray films and CT scan film, along with the orders for a direct admission to the oncology unit.

When the oncologist came in after looking at the films, he sat down with us and asked us, "What do you want for us to do? This is an aggressive cancer, and I can't promise that we can get you out of this crisis. We also can't promise much hope with chemo. And, if we do start the chemo, it is going to be very rough riding."

My brother looked at him, then at me, and said, "If we don't start something soon, especially the radiation, this tumor is going to choke me to death. I'd like to at least try."

A flurry of activity began after the doctor left the room. The radiation oncologist came up and talked and then he was taken downstairs for "markings" for the radiation.

The chemo began the next morning after the first radiation treatment. There would be thirty-three of them. He was still coughing up blood and something that looked like a small piece of his liver.

While I was out for a bathroom break I called Dad, my siblings, and my aunt and uncle, who are so close to us kids. But Jeffrey wasn't in the mood for company, so they came in for a brief visit and then all went to the waiting room area next to the elevators. It was good to see all of them; their presence strengthened me. I called my patient husband and told him I didn't know when I would be home.

The next day he felt more like having some company so Uncle Red drove up to give me a brief break. He and Jeffrey were always teasing each other before this and they decided not to change that. Jeffrey told him, "Listen, I've made Aunt Chris the president of this 'helping fetch me things' while I'm here, and you can be the vice-president. Right now I need some coffee." Off Uncle Red ran to the coffee pot, lickity split, to retrieve the request. He brought back caffeine-free coffee with cream. My brother said, "Well, you must be demoted to an aide. I want it straight, and with no cream. You have one more chance!"

We all were laughing and it felt so good. Uncle Red would have fetched the moon and stars if Jeffrey would have asked.

It was just so much so quickly that absorbing all of it was more than he had realized. He needed me close by, he said, but he needed some privacy at the same time and getting any privacy in a hospital is a joke. Still he told me he was so thankful to be there and getting the chemo and radiation, as hard and uncomfortable as it was; it was a gift, in a sense.

So, I told him I was going to the cafeteria for some soup and that I would be right back, which gave him a few moments. And I was able to hide in a bathroom far away from anyone who knew me and cry and scream into my jacket. All I could pray was, "Please, God, help us. Please give him some more time. Please help me to be strong and not show weakness in front of him."

The chemo lived up to its reputation. We were up and down all night with him vomiting and moaning; then there were more IV fluids and more IV antibiotics. He continued to cough up blood. But the nurses helped us and they gave him some IV pain medication. He kept doing his best to fight.

I was on the visitors' couch watching him as he finally drifted off to sleep again. I was aware that I was breathing in short, shallow breaths and took a quiet, deep breath and fell into a deep sleep. I was dreaming that I was trying to save him as a child from one episode after another. I was trying to grab a hold of his arm and pull him out of a deep pit and I couldn't quite firm up that grip, and he was slipping out of my reach.

When I jerked awake I looked at him and he was still asleep. I didn't want to go back to sleep. I started talking to myself: "He's right here. You are right here. You are protecting him now. You're helping him with all you can bring his way. He is safe for now."

The radiation team was so very compassionate and he was feeling better as we made our way with him on the gurney being pushing by a very young-looking orderly chewing gum and listening to his iPod in one ear. My brother was rolling his eyes but smiling. He was honestly excited about getting the radiation started.

As they rolled him away to have that first dose, I thought, "Who are you, brother of mine, you of so much courage?"

I was taken away by a memory of visiting him in a hospital several years before that when he had been admitted from a broken eye socket from a man beating him nearly to death with brass knuckles for being late on a loan. It was so unreal to me that anyone could do that. Jeffrey answered my disbelief, "That's what he gets paid very well to do. It happens."

He asked for no pity. But I could see that Dad was more troubled than the rest of us. My brother looked at him and said, "Don't do anything stupid."

Jeffrey was such a flirt when he felt well. And I guess with the excitement of getting to start this (death reprieve) radiation was pulling up the old charm out of him. He was flirting with those girls back there like he was twenty years old. And, bless them, they were laughing and going on with him like they all might go out later for cokes and hot dogs at the local Dairy Delight.

I wanted to run up and hug their necks, but I pretended not to notice his antics. It was like a ray of sunshine right before black clouds reached us.

After ten days of being in the hospital, the first few rounds of chemo done and ten days of radiation, we headed home. He was not coughing up blood anymore, he didn't have a fever, and he wasn't nauseated. He was more than ready to get out of there.

The best gift he had received in so long was waiting for him at Dad's house. Mallarie, his daughter, and her three little ones and Jeffrey's ex-wife and her boyfriend had arrived at the house. They lived in Kansas and had made the trip so they could see him and so he could see them. I have never seen him so excited in his whole life. They were going to get to stay the whole weekend.

Dad was so giving. He moved out to the travel trailer and let them have the whole house. I excused myself after hugging everyone and went over the chemo precautions and medication schedule and importance of hydration. Then I high-tailed it out of there to my home and my hubby.

When I went to pick him up for the drive back for his next radiation treatment, he was chatting about how much fun they had and that they didn't even make him nervous too much and that it was good to see his ex-wife and that he liked her boyfriend and on and on and on....

"Thank you, God; thank you, God!" I was reciting to myself in my head with another ray of sunshine!

Then on the way to the hospital, he turned to me and said, "I nearly died at the house that night a couple of weeks ago."

I didn't even look his way and spouted out, "No kidding! You were purple when I got there!"

He started again, "No, Becki, I'm serious. I nearly died."

I turned to look at him this time and, because of years of caring for terminally ill patients, I asked him, "What did you see?"

He said, "Well, when I was choking, all of a sudden I was surrounded by peace and quiet and on either side of me was Mom and my friend who committed suicide a few years ago. And I was pleading with them, 'Not yet, please, not yet.'

"And then Mom said, 'Then breathe Jeffrey, breathe.' And I was choking again, and then Dad was holding me up and shaking me. I think it was really them."

"Oh, Jeffrey, what a gift she gave you! Again, you've been given more time." And we drove the rest of that hour to the hospital without saying much at all.

Once they rolled him back into the treatment room, I hurried outside and called my siblings. They were speechless.

I just have no idea how that works. I can't explain it, but anytime any patient has ever told me that they saw family members that had passed years before come visit them, I never took it lightly. I never told them they were just dreaming. I listened and respected the honor that they were able to share it with me.

Thanks, Mom.

The longer the radiation continued—and especially on the days when we had to also drive over to the oncologist office and get his chemo—the harder it was for Jeffrey to feel up to talking or up to forcing food down or finding anything good to watch on television.

But the great gifts he received from time to time were phone calls from some of his buddies in Ponca City, the AA crowd. Oh, how they loved him. They gave him reminders that only they could give, and they made him laugh with memories than only they could share. I'll forever be grateful for what they did for him.

On one visit to the hospital radiation department, we were out in the waiting room and he struck up a conversation with an older gentleman, and they started talking about welding and construction and were in their own little world. I scooted over to the table with a *People* magazine and tried to find interest in a celebrity's messed-up life. I was pitiful and without compassion for the celebrity that day. "Loser," I thought.

And I found that all of my pain and emotion and fear were coming out in surprising ways. Once I felt like punching a rude customer in Wal-mart, but stopped myself, realizing they could sit on me and I would never have gotten a good shot.

Another time I was feeding the birds and I sat down on the ground out behind our house and fell over crying about how pretty the view was. My husband said I needed a real nap.

But I did not let my defenses down. I was in battle mode; I had to stay in battle mode, didn't I?

When we made our visits to the oncologist's office for outpatient chemotherapy Jeffrey tried to be very pleasant with the nurses, and he had compassion for those lined up in the recliners in that room. One day he walked in and asked an older gentleman, "Hey, buddy, how you doing?"

"Well, it's a damn party is what it is in this joint!" he replied.

Everyone in that room started laughing. It was a great way to start the chemo that day. I felt myself breathe a less frightful breath.

"Thank you, God."

After so many chemo treatments he was sent to the place where they do scans to see if the chemo is working. We did that one day and then headed to a Burger King because he felt like he could eat a cheeseburger and fries and a wanted to try to drink a Dr. Pepper. So while he is chowing down on this food, I got a call from the oncologist's nurse. "Becki, the report is in from the scan, and the doctor believes that the tumor has significantly shrunk to almost nothing!"

Oh! I can't even begin to tell you how liberating that news was to us. Jeffrey kept saying, "What did she say?" We were cautious but thrilled. We called everyone we knew who was praying or had put him on their church prayer lists. We were giddy, cautiously giddy. It was his birthday, number fifty-two, and what a nice gift.

The oncologist said we had to switch him to a different chemo since he took all he could take of the last one. So next visit he started him on a new one. Jeffrey was so eager, even after hearing the side effects.

One evening he called me and his temperature was 104. An infection can kill you when you're on chemo and your immune system is so compromised. He knew this and was trying so hard to live that he agreed going to the hospital for evaluation and IV antibiotics. But he didn't like it one bit. He was not very nice to the nurses or the lab personnel and was close to disowning me as well. Dad stayed out in the hallway. He wanted to be nearby but not too close. My brother didn't want any visitors during that hospitalization.

I was so tired that I was cranky as well and had to hide from him that I wanted him to shut up being so rude to people who were trying to help him. Yes, I understood that he didn't feel well and wasn't himself and was scared silly, but so was I. But then I started crying in my car that I was thinking such thoughts!

After about five days, he was discharged and that made him nicer. And we began the trips back to the outpatient oncology office for more good-and-bad, cell-killing chemo. But he did not shrink from the task before him. He even went back to flirting with the nurses.

After so many weeks of this particular chemo it was time for another scan. But it was close to Christmas and that scan was scheduled after the first of the year.

He asked me if I would buy a small Christmas tree so we could put it in the living room by the TV. It was only about three or four feet tall, fake but not too bad looking. I bought a couple of strings of lights, small multicolored bulbs, some silver tinsel, and an angel to put on top. We turned on an old Christmas movie while we decorated the tree. Mom used to love Christmas and always played Bing Crosby's "White Christmas" when we were kids. She would bake cookies and cut snowflakes out of our school papers to put on the windows. We didn't have much in the way of material gifts, but we had some great memories of going to Grandma and Grandpa's for Christmas Eve dinner with the whole family and then unwrapping gifts. So we talked about that for a while.

"Turn off that lamp and let me see what it looks like in the dark," he asked as he made his way back to his recliner.

"Well," he said, "isn't she a pretty little tree! Thank you for doing this."

I forgave all the rest when he said things like that. I could not save him, but I could put up a little tree for him!

So after the first of the year we headed back to the hospital for the scan and waited with abundant anxiety for the results, hoping that maybe, just maybe, we would have a cure.

Not so.

It was so heartbreaking when we were sitting in the oncologist's office and he had to tell us the tumor was growing again, so we needed to switch to another chemo. The doctor asked him if he wanted to continue trying. "Yes. Anything we can do to keep fighting."

We didn't talk much on that trip home. He pulled out a few AA lines though: "It is what it is." That's the one I remembered while driving to my house after getting him home, gripping the steering wheel like I was trying to squeeze blood out of it.

We started the new chemo on a day that was so cold I hated to have to drag him outside to get into the car. I hated to have him get out in the cold to go into the oncology office. But he acted like it was a gift: another chance that he didn't want to spoil with complaining about the cold. He was almost upbeat. While parking the car and pulling on my hat and gloves I prayed, "Please, God, he wants just a little more time."

While he was getting his treatment I walked to the car to retrieve a book I might read. Then I began wondering if I could ever write about all of this. It was too raw, all my journaling, too raw to print. There were so many words, thoughts, and emotions, like little scraps of paper with scribbling on them floating around in my head. But when I tried to organize them, tidy them up...I scream in my head, "NO, NOT YET!" We were still going to see the oncologist and getting the radiation treatments, and the lab, and talking to DHS and Social Security. So I kept those little floating scraps thrown, strewn across the floor of my brain, for safekeeping to collect later.

I could hear myself, "The Keeper must be strong, calm, clear, and focused. She cannot fall apart with preparatory grief or fear of the future. Just do today. Make the phone calls, go to the lab, schedule the surgeon's visit for the infusaport placement, secure financial breathing space, observe and respond accordingly to siblings, to Dad. Walk, meditate, pray, read, and yes, express to really safe friends a tiny bit of the raw, "He is my brother. I've always been the big sister. I cannot fix this. I cannot spare him what lies ahead, or my sisters, or Dad. They will listen and nod. They do not judge."

This is what I do. This is who I am. This is my life on purpose, caring, listening, supporting, teaching, learning, and being "present." I can't bake a pie to help. He's not hungry anyway. He marches into the oncology office with such bravery and flirts with his nurses, all 127 pounds of him. Thank heavens my sisters did know how to bring creature comforts. One would trim his hair or take him for a ride to The Dutch Pantry and treat him to a bite of something he might think he could eat and the other one would come and visit and let him talk and talk. He loved them dearly for their attempts, their time and their gifts.

Now it was February. He wanted to live, even though IT was creeping around outside the original limits seeking new blood supply, stealing his appetite, his desire to go out. He loaded up in my VW Rabbit without complaint to do whatever the doctor said we must do to keep up the fight...for how long?

"I just want to do it right." Those are the words in my head. Why? There's no grading scale. Who says it's right or wrong? A-minus or B-plus??

His favorite oncology nurse was as chipper as ever. She never, ever let on like there was any bad news being delivered in any of those rooms. Her positive attitude and upbeat demeanor, I think, was one of the reasons she was his favorite.

Spring was so welcomed. As soon as daytime was warm and safe enough, we got out the lawn chairs and sat on the front porch area for him to look at the pasture to the south and smell the air and feel the sunshine on his bald head. He didn't weigh much over 100 pounds by then, but he didn't care: he was fighting and when he got a chance later, perhaps, he would eat more. He just wanted to be outside. He missed the old welding days and being out all the time, rain or shine, hot or cold. He used to tell me about one of his favorite coastlines and all the sightseeing on his days off and the history of some of the towns.

He was so smart; no one ever told him that. He was told he was NOT very smart since he couldn't read very well and since he was held back in the first grade and so on and so on. He watched a lot of the History Channel and would tell me all he had learned and he would watch the Discovery Channel and the National Geographic Channel. For relaxation he would watch the channel where they were showing car repairs, antique car auctions, and a little NASCAR. Oh, how thankful I was for this. He escaped for thirty minutes to an hour at times away from the looming cloud.

His lung cancer was now in Stage 4 and progressing. It had spread to his middle chest area and other spots in his right lung. He was to start a "milder" chemo to help slow this progression down on March 11 but on the tenth he was admitted to the hospital with a collapsed left lung, possibly due to the infusaport insertion into his left chest the week before. But he improved, the chest tube was removed, and in four days he returned home. He was proud he had gained some weight, 112 pounds. Chemo would begin March 26.

Now nearing early summer, it was time for another scan. We went to the little room they escorted us to, to wait for the doctor and the results of that scan. His favorite nurse came in with him and wasn't her cheerful self. My heart sank. The doctor arrived.

"Mr. Charles, I'm afraid the chemo isn't working. It's time to stop. Also the lab work shows that your hepatitis has returned."

"Can we try another drug? Can we go back to that first chemo that helped the most? Can I go back to the liver doctor and see if I can take that hepatitis medicine again?" he earnestly asked.

I was dying listening to him.

The doctor shook his head, "I'm sorry, but no. It's just time to quit now. We will keep you as much pain-free as possible. We can start hospice and I know your sisters and dad will help you."

The nurse came over and patted his shoulder. My brother got up and said, "Well, I want to thank you for trying. I've had longer than I thought I would. How long do you think I have?"

"Weeks."

I didn't want to further upset him by saying anything he didn't want to hear so I was keeping my mouth shut.

He said, "One day at a time, Becki, one day at a time."

I decided to tell Dad in person and, I have to say, that was one of the hardest things I have ever done in my life.

Then I called our siblings and other relatives and asked them to continuing praying for all of us. We're related to great prayer warriors.

Hospice. It's what I knew best. I called the local hospice group that I used to work for and asked for their help and for them to come evaluate, among other things. They were very kind and reminded me to try to be just a sister and not a nurse. Yeah, right.

I waited until he was ready for me to call them. He said he didn't want a hospital bed yet and he just mainly wanted them to be there if we needed them.

We were trying to let him have as much control as possible. And yet that domineering, older sister, nurse person that I was kept trying to be in control and make sure everything was being offered; I was always, always, trying to protect him. But he was, never being the dummy, aware and was open and honest with me. "I totally understand where we are at this point. All of the family can rest assured that me and God are good. I have made peace with everyone I had hoped to make peace with."

"Okay. I'll try then not to be so bossy and try to run the show. It's your show. But I was wondering, do you have any questions?" I asked holding my breath again.

"No. I've researched this enough on my laptop, and I've figured out just about how this is going to go. I just want you to stay on top of making sure they keep me medicated for pain as much as you can."

I was pulling up in the driveway at Dad's house one day for a visit when I noticed Jeffrey was sitting in his truck. I wasn't even sure how he got in it. I approached carefully so as not to surprise him.

"Hey, whatcha doin'?"

"I'm going to town. I want to go to Sonic and get a corndog and tater tots and maybe a Coke." He answered still facing the windshield.

"Well, my car is parked behind your truck. Can I drive you? I'd like to get a grilled cheese," I asked hoping he would agree.

"Yeah, that would be all right," he said.

So we drove to town and right to the Sonic and I ordered our food. He carefully put mustard and ketchup on his corndog and some on his tater tots and took one bite. Then he wadded it all up in the paper bag and handed it to me. He didn't say a word.

I got Jeffrey home and he asked to sit on the front porch. He was weak and trembling. "How long do you think I have? I was thinking maybe a couple of months," he asked while looking out at the pasture.

"Well, I think a couple of months might be a little generous, but you never know."

He stood up and I made it to him before he fell. I got him in the house. How we made it up those steps can only be defined as a miracle. I didn't want to take him to the hospital with broken bones.

He agreed to let me have hospice bring the bed BUT, he said, he was the one who would decide when he needed to be in it. For now he wanted to stay in his recliner. I didn't argue and I didn't agree that day. I knew the day would come soon enough to insist he not get out of the bed without help.

For Father's Day our two other sisters came over with their mates and we fixed some food and gave Daddy his gifts. My brother's pain med was helping with the pain, but decreasing his ability to motivate safely. The family gathered in the kitchen while the hospice nurse assessed him and the aide helped him with a sponge bath and shave. He was now officially a skeleton with skin, a hospital gown, glasses, and dentures, and don't forget determined (yet) spirit.

I have the photo of that day where we three girls are gathered around the head of his bed and we are all smiling. How did we do that? He had just looked out the north living room window and said, "I think I'm having a hallucination. I just saw Dad's head pass by without his body." We started laughing and told him that Daddy was mowing the lawn right next to the window.

"Oh, good," he said, "I thought I was worse off than I realized."

That's when my brother-in-law snapped the photo.

In the photo he's still unconvinced and looking out the window smiling, and the three of us are laughing one last time.

One evening Dad called me and said, "Becki, I don't think I can do this anymore by myself, without someone else here to help me watch over him all night long. I'm afraid I'll not give that pain medicine right."

I moved in with them for the duration. I still didn't know how long he had. His vital signs were still strong, but he wasn't eating or drinking much at all. He was having some increase in his confusion due to the disease process and the pain medication and, of course, trouble breathing as well.

I slept on the couch facing his bed. I lay there watching him breathe and listening for any moaning that usually started when the pain med was wearing off. Trying to stay ahead of that game was challenging. Enough...not too much...but now not enough...just a little more...that's better.

I'm a firm believer that prayers from family and friends are what kept me from dying from fatigue and grief. Our two sisters were so supportive and would come as often as they could. Sheer will played a huge part in it as well. I slept with fitful dreams and one eye always open.

The night before he passed, he sat up in his bed and turned to look at me and smiled. "Oh, I'm glad you are here. My sister is a nurse."

I smiled and returned, "That's nice. Yes, I'm staying the night with you. You can go back to sleep."

He lay back down and looked at me for another minute or so and smiled again. Then we went back to sleep. Sort of.

That last night we were up all night. He could not get comfortable. I tried everything. I had given the medication for sleep and anxiety and respiratory distress but still he was fighting and fighting. At one point I woke up Dad and asked him to help me turn him to another position to see if it would help. It did but only for a few minutes.

Dad sat in his recliner and rocked and rocked.

My brother started moaning and we decided to try to turn him and reposition his pillow while I continually talked softly to him reminding him we were with him and we would not leave him. As Dad sat back down, Jeffrey quit breathing. I motioned Dad to come.

"Daddy, he's going now."

"Oh, Jeffy, oh son, I love you," he said.

210

"It's okay, brother, go to the Light; Mom is waiting. We love you."
It was over.

A surge of relief flooded me before the grief. I glanced at the clock for the time. I held my Dad and let him cry. Then he went to the kitchen to make coffee. I called the hospice nurse and the funeral home.

"Thank you, God; he's not suffering anymore," was what I was praying. Then I noticed I was breathing somewhat normal again.

He had told me a few weeks before that he wanted to be cremated and he didn't care what I did with the ashes. I cared.

I didn't cry until my husband walked in the door. I soaked his shirt as he held me.

"He's safe now. I don't have to try to protect him anymore. He's okay. He's with God and Mom and Grandma and Grandpa and Uncle Rod and Aunt Bea and his friend that died and all the others."

Only one more promise to fulfill: the service.

I think I was still in a fatigue/shock/relief state of mind as I wrote out the funeral service and picked the songs with my siblings' agreement. Friends from his Ponca City AA group sent flowers and lovely written words about what he meant to them and what he had done for the city of Ponca by speaking to the high school teens about the dangers of drugs and alcohol.

I pieced together all these tributes and with all the gumption I could gather up started writing about Jeffrey.

Again, I know without a doubt that it was God's grace and mercy to me from all those prayers holding me up to give me the strength to get up there and lead that service.

I keep his ashes in my office where I write and pray and read and meditate.

My brother's keeper?
Yes.

EPILOGUE

So what are the most important lessons I've learned from my patients? We are beautiful beloved souls, one human family, who for a brief time, even if you live to be 110, are here to learn how to love one another unconditionally and to love God—All That Is, Spirit, whatever you choose to call the Higher Power—with all that we are.

One dear lady said, "Becki, this is Earth School. We are learning from these joys and from these diversities, these days of sunshine and of rain to grow our souls. We 'flesh out' the meaning of how we love our God by how we love one another."

They teach me to learn the beauty of just being present to one another in our dying journey and that we can still celebrate life until the moment we die.

They speak words of wisdom to all of us if we listen. When they are communicating regrets, listen. When they are remembering love in their life, listen. When they are releasing anger, listen. When they speak of angels or loved ones arriving days or hours before they are leaving us, we can humbly bow in honor of the hour and the holy ground. What a privilege it is to be with them.

They remind me that if I am visiting them, whether climbing up their entrance of marble steps to a mansion or concrete blocks to a mobile home, that we are all the same in those hours. Our needs are truly the same, universally: Will you sit with me? Will you hear me? How will you help me with my discomfort, my emotional, my spiritual, my physical pain?

They teach me to remember that the only thing we take with us is the Love woven into the fabric of our souls. Not the bank account, not the jewels, not the awards. Truly, at the end of the day, all that really matters is how we treat one another.

The underlining theme is Unconditional Love.

It is my prayer for you that as you continue your journey you KNOW this love and that you GIVE your love freely, unconditionally. I also pray that when your time comes to Transition, there will be someone at your side to remind you how precious and beloved you are, someone who will sing or tell funny stories, or read your favorite book, or sit silently and hold your hand, reminding you of what a gift you have been to this space and place called Life.

Know that you are never alone.

In Love and Light,

Becki

APPENDIX

HOW TO BE PRESENT TO OUR LOVED ONES IN TRANSITION

HOW TO 'BE PRESENT' TO THE DYING

"Becki, how on earth am I going to know what to do or say when I visit my friend, Bill? He is in the last stages of his cancer. His wife called and said Bill would like to see me again. I don't know what to say. And I'm afraid if I do say something, it'll be wrong.

Many people have asked me these types of questions. My patients and their loved ones helped me learn how to 'be with' their mother, father, child, spouse, or friend...whoever it was I was visiting. They taught me to take cues from the ones who were primary caregivers in the home and the patient as well. Sometimes it's our presence more than what we say.

The majority of the ones I've visited were not into long visits and were not into too much chattering. They seemed to always appreciate knowing ahead of time if you were coming to visit. They liked having as much control for as long as possible. If they were having difficulty getting their pain under control one afternoon, it'd be better to come another day.

Be sensitive to the big picture. Are they tired from too much company? Did they have a sleepless night? It's always a good idea to visit with the caregivers and ask their opinion on when to visit. But keep it short. More than once I've visited a patient and they would say something like, "My next door neighbor Sue came over and stayed over an hour talking about everyone on our block. I didn't think she'd ever leave."

If you are a very close friend it is usually a good idea to visit about what you have always talked about. Did you watch football together? Did you golf together? Did you go shopping together? You could briefly touch on what you have in common.

I observed one dear fellow who was visiting his best friend. He was honest right away. "Sam, I just wanted you to know I'm praying for you and I don't have a clue what to say right now. I mainly wanted you to know that I care." His friend smiled and replied, "Hank, don't worry about that. We are both new to this. I don't know what to say either. I feel like I might be able to watch part of that TU basketball game if you'd like to sit with me." From that day forward they just eased into being able to talk about what seemed natural to them. When Hank would notice Sam nodding off, he'd quietly excuse himself and return home.

Where one personality will share with you all that's on their heart, another one will rarely say a word, but both appreciate the gesture of the visit.

I'm still learning after thirty years. I will say that they have told me many times that "showing up" is the most important thing anyone can say or do. Even if you realize immediately that another day would be better, your action of taking time to be brave enough to stop by speaks volumes.

Bless you for caring enough to conquer your fear of going to see your friend or loved one. One fellow said to me after a few questions, "I'd hope someone would visit me!"

HOW TO SIT WITH THOSE WHO ARE GRIEVING

I am also frequently asked by friends, relatives, and acquaintances about how to "visit" the ones who are grieving. "Becki, what am I supposed to say?" "What if I say the wrong thing?" "How long should I visit?" "Should I offer to do something?" These are examples of some of the questions that come to me.

So what do we say? The number one answer I get from grieving loved ones is that there isn't anything that really sounds great, but that "I'm so genuinely sorry," isn't as insulting or rude or unkind.

Being present with someone who is grieving speaks volumes. Be sensitive to not staying too long. Listening is one of the best ways to express our love for one another. And yes, check with the family or primary spokesperson for the family about anything you might be able to do: run an errand, mow the lawn, walk the dog, get the oil changed in the car, do a load of laundry...whoever is attending the one grieving will let you know. And sometimes we can observe an obvious need and just do it.

I don't pretend to be an authority in this. I am just sharing what thirty years of being with these dear ones has helped me to learn by their voices. Bless you for wanting to help in any way. For as we all know all too well, one day it will be us.

There are all kinds of books, pamphlets, articles on grief. Google the word "grief" and you will find one you are more comfortable with than others. It's good to do a little research. There are books for children grieving, books for those who lost a child to suicide, violent death...a wide range of grieving self-help, etc.

Some of my favorite books are:

- A set of booklets by Kenneth C. Haugk, "Journeying through Grief"
- *Good Grief* by Granger E. Westberg
- *After Goodbye* by Ted Menten
- *Grieving, A Love Story* by Ruth Coughlin
- *On Grief and Grieving* by Elizabeth Kubler-Ross, David Kessler